Hoverboard

Make Money Selling & Repairing Hoverboards

(Profiting From This Modern Day Hoverboard Gold Rush)

Jennie Roberts

Published By **Elena Holly**

Jennie Roberts

All Rights Reserved

Hoverboard: Make Money Selling & Repairing Hoverboards (Profiting From This Modern Day Hoverboard Gold Rush)

ISBN 978-1-77485-454-9

All rights reserved. No part of this guide may be reproduced in any form without permission in writing from the publisher except in the case of brief quotations embodied in critical articles or reviews.

Legal & Disclaimer

The information contained in this book is not designed to replace or take the place of any form of medicine or professional medical advice. The information in this book has been provided for educational and entertainment purposes only.

The information contained in this book has been compiled from sources deemed reliable, and it is accurate to the best of the Author's knowledge; however, the Author cannot guarantee its accuracy and validity and cannot be held liable for any errors or omissions. Changes are periodically made to this book. You must consult your doctor or get professional medical advice before using any of the suggested remedies, techniques, or information in this book.

Upon using the information contained in this book, you agree to hold harmless the Author from and against any damages, costs, and expenses, including any legal fees potentially resulting from the application of any of the information provided by this guide. This disclaimer applies to any damages or injury caused by the use and application, whether directly or indirectly, of any advice or information presented, whether for breach of contract, tort, negligence, personal injury, criminal intent, or under any other cause of action.

You agree to accept all risks of using the information presented inside this book. You need to consult a professional medical practitioner in order to ensure you are both able and healthy enough to participate in this program.

Table Of Contents

Introduction 1

Chapter 1: A Beginning Of The Hoverboard 4

Chapter 2: Boards 101 12

Chapter 3: Business 23

Chapter 4: Suppliers And Purchasing Your Inventory 41

Chapter 5: Liability Beware Of Scams And Losses 49

Chapter 6: What To Sell 64

Chapter 7: The Hoverboard Manual 74

Chapter 8: Advantages And Use Of Self-Balancing Electronic Scooters And Electronic Hoverboards 93

Chapter 9: Drop Shipping 108

Chapter 10: Today! 117

Chapter 11: Hover Or Glide 119

Chapter 12: Inside Out 122

Chapter 13: Accessories 128

Chapter 14: The Reality Of Fantasy 131
Chapter 15: Motivation 137
Chapter 16: Self-Talk 172

Introduction

If you've tried wholesale, e-commerce, or drop-shipping previously or if this is the first time you've tried it you're taking this course, this comprehensive course will teach you everything you'll ever require or need to learn about the best way you can begin an Hoverboard business.

In the six months leading up to Christmas, I earned more than $25,000 from selling scooters that self-balance themselves which isn't even my main business. This is a side business for me. Hoverboards were the most sought-after present for Christmas in 2015. Gift in 2015.

Although they've been on the west coast in 2015, they're just getting bigger, excuse the pun, all over the nation with millions of people purchasing hoverboards. The market isn't overcrowded and is likely to keep growing.

Alongside Hoverboards the whole "ride-able device" sector is growing. This encompasses everything from one-wheel skateboards, electric bikes, one wheel motorcycles and with new and innovative devices appearing every day, which opens up even more possibilities.

If you're skeptical about the popularity of these hoverboards, as well as the entire industry I would like to challenge you to look up something like Google Trends, Google Keyword Planner or Terapeak to determine how many searches per month are being performed for hoverboards as well as the number that are being sold.

We'll examine this from a variety of perspectives. If you don't wish to keep inventory, or do not have the funds to invest in it We'll discuss ways to go about this via drop shipping. Another method that requires no beginning expenditure is affiliate marketing.

For those who prefer to keep your own inventory but aren't willing to pay hundreds of thousands of dollars to be able to do so We'll talk about the best way to run this business by examining the e-commerce angle and retail.

For those who are willing to invest some more money into this project, you are able to look into imports and/or wholesaling.

This program will discuss not only selling boards as well as selling components that can be used to repair boards as well as for those who are tech-savvy and/or handy, fixing them also. There is a lot of money to be made in Hoverboard Repairs.

Chapter 1: A Beginning Of The Hoverboard

Who would have imagined that a film would kick off with a race of this kind? "The big-budget Trilogy movies "Back to the Future "sparked the imagination of many viewers in "Back to the Future, Part II" in which Marty McFly stepped on the hoverboard in the future" 2015 of the skateboards that would be. In the sequel we saw the hoverboard on the screen as part of "Back to the Future, Part Three." It's true Director Robert Zemeckis played this up by teasing the viewers with an idea of the hoverboard's existence. (SEITZ, 2014)

But, who thought it up? The co-author Bob Gale from the movie confesses that this idea was conceived" within a basement, while considering the scene from the skateboarding Marty who was running across Biffs" vehicle to the skateboard he would similar to in 2015. (Gale 2015) For some the idea was a amazing idea, but to others, it was a way to ignited their imagination. And then there were those who had to figure out an approach to attempt the impossible. The impossible isn"t at all impossible in the end.

History
1900's

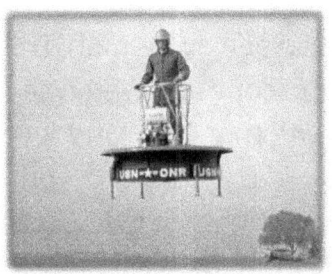

It is the U.S. Navy
As of 1955, the world had an aircraft platform that could fly. A manufacturer of aircrafts that was shown by the Navy created it. (Hover Past, 2015) The Army was able to stop it as they thought it was tiny, unstable and not able to reach higher above the ground. It would have been nice if they knew the extent of what they were committing to! What would we'd see today? The vehicle they used was opposite-rotating air-powered fans, powered through direct-lift rotors.

The pilot would stand on the platformand controlling it using his weight, and then move in the direction he desired to move.

2000-2013

Dean Kamen

in 2001 Dean Kamen brought us his creation in 2001, the Segway Human Transporter. It had five gyroscopes as well as an integrated computer in the first models. In 2003, consumers was able to purchase the Segway. While the Segway was equipped with handles but the technology was based on shifting of the weight of the user and the an adjustable handlebar that could be manually turned. The Segway had three versions available at the time.

In light of their weight and how heavy they were, they were priced at $3000.00. (Bellis) In the year 2006 Kamen discontinued production these models and introduced two new models that permitted the steering to lean instead of manual turning.

Jamie Hyneman

Jamie Hyneman, of Myth Busters fame has tried his hand at creating a hoverboard for the show, using the surfboard and a leaf blower. He gave it the name of"the

"Hyneman Hoverboard" and it appeared it would outdo Adam"s quite a large version of an advertisement in an old magazine that stated, "Anyone could create an alternative technology at their own home, away from large businesses and the government." They made use of common household items to construct their hoverboards. Jamie"s boards, to say the a minimum appeared to be one, though he seemed to be somewhat too confident with the motors for leaf blowers compared to Adam"s cleaning machine motors.

It was really enjoyable to watch, however both players looked exhausted (not to the teams)! They seemed to be working more hard to determine who would win the game! They were all exhausted when the contest was finished. The legend? It was plausible but not feasible!

Jason Bradbury

The year 2005 was the first time The Gadget Show TV presenter from Brittian has experimented in the concept of building the hoverboard. He built a wooden platform as well as an air blower. He attempted to do it again in 2009, but this time with the jet engine. (Graham Parish Engineering, 2009)

Nils Guadagnin

French musician Nils Guadagnin created an electronic hoverboard in 2011, which employed magnetic aversion. Its drawback was that it wasn't capable of supporting the weight. It can also lift itself by means of the electromagnetic field. Nils" idea when he created this model from"Back To The Future "Back to the Future" Part II" Overboard, was that it would give sculptures a sense of spatiality. (GUADAGNIN, 2010)

Universite Paris Diderot

Researchers from the Universite Paris Diderot created an ultraconductor skateboard at the Materials and Quantum Phenomena Laboratory. The skateboard runs along a magnetic track. all you need to do is get onto the board. It's referred to as"the Mag Surf, and it is able to travel on the magnetic track around two inches above the surface. The use of liquid nitrogen can make the iron at the bottom of the board cold, which allows it to transform into superconductor. (Smalley 2011) Overall, we're getting close, don"t you think?

2013

Smart S1 or HoverTrax

There are many locations to purchase these two-wheeled marvels. As per David Pierce of Wired, (PIERCE, 2015)Prices range is extremely in many instances. It's like they're made out of gold! There are various sizes of colors and variations in shape. Are they all alike? No. The company that claims that it has the patent(s) are Hangzhou Chic Intelligent Technology Co., Ltd., but there's an issue with this. It appears that Shane Chen has a patent (2014). According to Joseph Bernstein, a BuzzFeed News Reporter thought, "...the so-called hoverboards could represent one of the Tickle Me Elmos of 2015... with one holiday season half-life." in his piece "The Hoverboard War" published September. 16, 2015 in the 5th minute of p.m. In any event I've heard of children who want hoverboards!

Yesteryear

It's not it was that long ago when we watched films that started the race to create the hoverboard. We've seen some interesting and interesting twists and turns in the course of development. In this article, we will examine what transpired in the year 2014, and we prepare to bid farewell to 2015.

I must say that 2014 was a very interesting year...

2014

HUVr

In March of 2014 HUVr was in prominence for only a short time. They claimed to have the technology behind the hoverboard. They also had major names of Tony Hawk, Terell Owens, Moby, and Christopher Lloyd himself in a commercial for their product via YouTube. Of of course, it was simple to determine the fact that this was an untrue ruse however, it left people in awe for a few minutes. It appears that people took it seriously, and there were big names involved. Lloyd. Lloyd felt bad and apologized for the prank. Thank you Monsieur. Lloyd! There were a few of us arrested! We were able to see the wires and the stuff.

Hendo Hover

October 2014 was when Greg Henderson, the American creator of Hendo Hover, created a prototype. However, there was some work to be completed before the device could be considered marketable. We know that they continue to work on it but there were just 10 such boards at the time, and they require an electrically conductive surface to use. There was speculation that Mr.

Henderson did not seem to be keen on the project Instead, he was looking to develop some sort of maglev emergency device. We're hoping that the Hendo Hover doesn"t abandon the project. We are hoping that Hendo Hover is really close to getting on the right path in this regard! (Sparkes, 2014)

Chapter 2: Boards 101

Hoverboards have been popular in the US since 2013. Take a look at Google trends and you'll notice increases in searches starting in 2013. The devices essentially died until 2015 when retailers and importers grew smarter and began giving free boards to famous people and YouTubers to help promote their products. The devices were then brought to the forefront and after that, sales began to increase.

Patents - Who owns Hoverboards?

There's plenty of contention regarding who is the owner of the rights to patents and Hoverboards. In the last year, Mark Cuban claimed to own the rights along with a co-partner of his who threatened to bring a lawsuit against Walmart should they sell the products.

I've had the pleasure of speaking with three other warehouse owners who showed me patent papers and claimed to have owned the warehouses.

Recently, Razor Scooter has claimed ownership, and is urging Amazon to block other sellers off of their platform.

The fact is that the patents are rather weak. They claim to patent the concept of a "two wheels rideable". My view is that this patent covers all the way from a bicycle to the original segway to a variety of other gadgets. Just changing the way that the device works or how it is built can be a sign that the seller isn't infringing the original patent.

I wouldn't be concerned or worried about this, but it's something you need to take note of.

Board Styles - Types Of Boards

In the past, there was one hoverboard available that is commonly referred to as"the first, traditional also known as a 6.5" board. They typically have 6.5" wheels that come in different colours. There are various variations that come with carrying handles wheel guards that cover them, as well as on the later models Bluetooth. These are typically the most popular and are generally the most affordable. According to my experience, they have less issues than the versions with 8" as well as the 10-" versions. The board can be seen in the picture below.

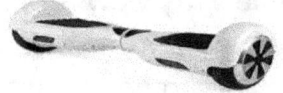

Eight" Boards are commonly known as the Lambo boards since it was designed on the Lambo Lamborghini. They're also referred to by the name of Diamond Boards due to the design of their platform. These boards usually come with LED lights on top of the wheels. They are also equipped with Bluetooth and usually keys fobs that can shut off the board and on, and then lock it. The boards I've had the highest number of returns on and the most problems have been with these eight" boards.

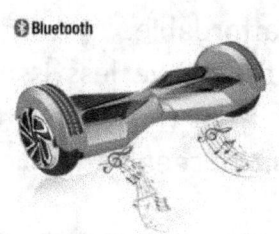

Then we can are also able to use"the 10" board that is often known as"the SUV" board. They usually have Bluetooth. Another thing that is different about these boards is that they feature the 10" inflating wheels. These boards generally ride better on rough and cracked surfaces. They also have more clearance to allow you to ride over rocks and small sticks without damaging the board.

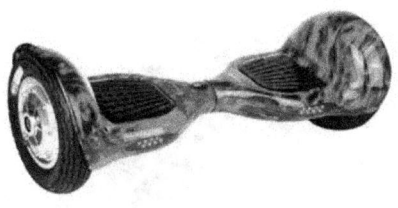

In recent times, some new styles of boards have come out like The Batman Board or X1. The basic idea is to have a different style from the other. Apart from these, we also have other ride-able gadgets such as the electric unicycle one wheel, which is a single wheel skateboard and a single wheel motorcycle. There are new inventions being developed each day. We won't go in detail about these devices however, take a look at the images in the gallery below...

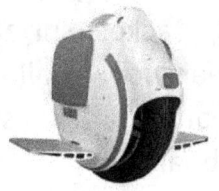

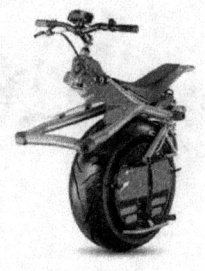

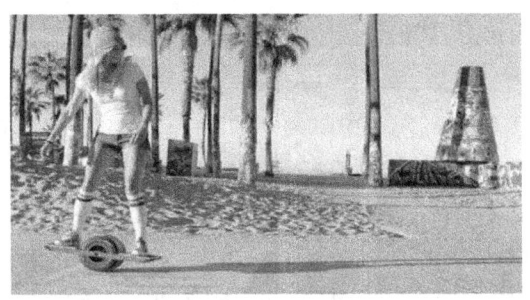

Safety

There's no doubt that you've been bombarded with the news of these hoverboards burning up or getting caught on fire. In reality, it's just hype and not the major issue it's being presented as. However, it's not a reason to not be careful, but thousands of boards were sold, and until now there's been around 9 fires.

There are even suggestions that the fires could be media manufactured by companies like ioHawk and others that sell higher priced boards. They are trying to convince the public that they should spend $1000 or more on an item instead of purchasing an "cheap" as well as "dangerous" board at a cost, like $200-$300.

Any device that is powered by an lithium ion battery is in the potential to explode.

Laptops, iPhones, cordless drills , and many other devices powered by batteries have seen their numbers explode, but we don't see anyone getting away with those devices. If you that you are aware of who you're purchasing from and what you're purchasing is, you will receive good quality batteries that are wired correctly and include fused connections and cutoffs that can prevent sparks and fires.

The best safety precautions include buying only high-quality boards, never charging your boards without monitoring and also not charging too much for your boards. Your customers should be encouraged to read the manual and adhere to these guidelines also.

Batteries

There's a lot of debate about batteries. There are many who have urged you to purchase boards that use Samsung and LG batteries. Samsung nor LG make Hoverboard batteries. They're not even made.

They do make cells that some sellers of hoverboards include in their batteries, however technically speaking, there isn't any such thing as the term "a Samsung or LG battery. The sellers can however utilize Samsung cell and LG Cells in the event that they design and put together battery packs for their products.

There are three kinds of batteries. There are those that contain Samsung cells, those that contain LG cells and "Chinese Battery". It is not necessary to worry about brand names, so long as you own an excellent and well-wired battery.

The batteries must have each individual cell wired individually instead of the entire 12 cells wired into one circuit, or perhaps 4 cells wired in three circuits. If all cell circuits are connected,, when one cell is damaged it will charge another cell in order to compensate. Overcharged or undercharged cells is not only harmful for the battery's health, but also poses risky for fire. If you examine the pictures above, the first photo shows an unwired battery. You can clearly see that, cells are wired in blocks of four, as opposed to being individual wires and monitored as shown in the picture below, which shows the white cells of the battery.

What Makes A Quality Board

What is it that makes a good board? Most boards are pretty identical and use similar parts. What differentiates them is the quality of components utilized. The quality of the assembly and the programing for the motherboard.

It is possible to hear that the board is very smooth to ride. Every board is programmed to perform in a particular way, at a particular speed, and to rotate in the same manner. Certain boards have their motherboards programmed better than others, and this can result in a more comfortable ride. Some boards are able to cut more efficiently or turn faster than others, based on how they are programmed. Certain boards can also be equipped with multiple speeds, such as the speed for training and speed for sports.

Before I purchase inventory, I usually purchase a few sample pieces. I'll then ride the board and then remove it from the board and inspect the interiors.

What I am looking for is how well the plastics and metals employed. I also consider how the board is constructed. Are all the screws utilized? In this case, for example the shell is fitted with 8 screws to secure it to its shell. The majority of boards have 4 screws. It's not an issue, but a board that has eight screws is a sign that the manufacturer doesn't want to save money or time by not putting in those additional screws which many factories aren't to put in.

The quality and fit in the finish of the shell are an additional sign. Certain boards have poor paint, whereas others sport an "new car" similar paint job, with the appearance of a clean and attractive shine. If the seller invests hours and efforts to make boards that are attractive and quality, it is likely that the interiors will be nicely constructed as well.

Before loading up any of the inventory, I'd suggest you purchase a few boards at different vendors, ride them before opening them up to take a look. Determine who has the highest quality board.

Another thing to be aware of, even for those who are planning on dropping-shipping but never handling the product, you should purchase an example piece to check out the board, so that you are sure you're selling a good product. Also, to give you an understanding of the product you are selling. At the time the client wants to get a refund, you are the person dealing with the issue and not dropping shippers.

Chapter 3: Business

In this article, we are going to look at the business aspect of selling hoverboards. Personally, I approached the issue in a variety of ways.

I began my career as an affiliate marketer, promoting hyperlinks that I was able to promote for Amazon, eBay, and Ali Express.

Then I moved to retail with a small-time focus. I bought a few boards from Ali Express and sold them locally through Craigslist or Offer Up. The first thing you'll notice is once you've established yourself as a seller of boards, you'll start receiving inquiries from wholesalers and importers you. When you're in the process suppliers will start coming to your door, and you'll be able to search for the lowest cost and conditions.

In this section , I'm going to provide greater detail about wholesale retail, drop-shipping selling parts, performing repairs, and much more.

Affiliate Marketing

I'm not going give you a complete instruction on how affiliate marketing works. market, but the idea is to make a promotion of an affiliate link or banner via your blog or social media channels, or through other methods.

As an affiliate, you receive specific links, which include an ID for tracking and a cookie. If someone clicks on your link and then is directed to a site such as Ali Express for example, they could purchase the item that you've connected them to.

If this happens, you receive an amount of cut or commission from the sales. In the case of Ali Express I was making commissions of 8 percent. On a typical $300 or $250 sale, I could earn between $20 and $30, which is a decent commission for an affiliate. It's better than earning $0.30 cents per click on Adsense.

In just one month, I earned more than $1000 selling hoverboards via Ali Express through Facebook, Twitter, Youtube videos, as well as other social media.

The way I achieved this was to provide useful content. I would provide reviews of hoverboards, create videos on hoverboards unboxing which I've had the greatest satisfaction with is videos on repair or tutorials on how to repair hoverboards.

They're especially useful when it comes to selling parts for repair. Many people aren't aware of how to fix a board therefore they search for videos about how to repair it. If you are able to identify their issue, demonstrate ways to repair it and offer the component they need and they are likely to purchase the part from you.

Drop Shipping

Drop shipping is the practice of selling products online that you don't own or have stocks of.

The following is basically drop-shipping in just a few words. I have found a company that can ship single boards to me to addresses of my clients. Drop shippers can perform what is known by the term "blind shipping". This means that the business is actually shipping the board but will not include packing slips , or packaging that displays their details and the buyer believes they're receiving the item from me.

There are people who use eBay, Amazon, or Ali Express for drop-shipping, but there are actually drop shippers who only order the fulfillment of other vendors. It's likely to be the best option because they are aware of what they do, and are able to create the illusion that the product is from you.

Here's how drop shipping is done. I locate my vendor. I build my website. After I get my first purchase for a green hoverboard , I orally submit an Excel form or contact my drop-shipper. I inform them that I want the green hoverboard to be delivered by Jim Smith in New York at his address.

I've already collected the funds from Jim I'll give him $400. I can purchase an item from my drop-shipper for just $200. I take Jim's payment through my website. Then, I call my dropshipper place my order and then pay them $200 to send this board directly to Jim.

I keep the difference of $200. If Jim decide to return the board, he'll return it via the drop shipping company, who is likely to charge me a re-stocking charge. If Jim decides to keep the board, I get my $200.

Before setting up drop shippers, I'd recommend purchasing a sample board to are aware of what your customers will receive and ensure that the quality is high.

A thing to be wary regarding is selling a low-quality product The drop shipper will take taken their money from you and you could be required to reimburse your client. Because drop shippers usually operate with smaller margins, this could result in a loss of cash if you are dealing with more than one return or issue.

Drop shipping is great as the drop shipper handles most of your work as well as because you do not have to carry physical items.

However, be aware that since you're purchasing individual pieces at once, for every customer, and also because your drop shipper does the majority of the work and you pay for it, you'll be paying more than if you purchased the physical items yourself in the bulk.

If you're in need of assistance with drop shipping, Shopify is the best option to start your store. They provide a range of useful applications and tools that can assist you in automatically integrating your drop shippers' product images and information and in certain cases, automatically transfer information about sales from your website onto your drop shipper. This basically simplifies the entire process for you.

E-commerce/Retail

This is a traditional method of business. You purchase inventory and own inventory. For instance, you purchase 50 hoverboards on a pallet.

As you buy in bulk you will get a fantastic price. We'll use $180 as an example. Then you can sell the hoverboards on your website or ebay, Amazon as well as locally through websites like Craigslist or Bookoo and apps such as 5 Miles or Offer Up.

The boards you purchase cost $180. You then sell them at $400, and keep the profits as well as the commission.

There are many methods to sell retail through online shopping. If you do not want to create the store yourself and manage your own traffic, or buy traffic from others, you could sell your products on eBay as well as Amazon.

If you're interested in creating your own online shop; Shopify, Big Commerce and GoDaddy offer great tools to set up an online store. It is not necessary to have technical knowledge of web design or programming There are a myriad of excellent apps for setting up referral programs and set up affiliate programs and get an entire army of associates for your business as we have described within the business plans for affiliate marketing.

There are many other excellent tools for managing the inventory, to up-sell customers at the end in your cart, and lots more.

If you want to set up an online store Mall kiosks are an excellent opportunity to sell. There's a lot of traffic, and is a good place to purchase an item on impulse such as a hoverboard.

If you or your friend are the owner of a mobile repair shop, it's a great spot to offer boards and components and an excellent method to enter the repair of hoverboards and.

Most cell phone shops have the tools and electronic expertise. This also aids in building confidence in the customer. The majority of people would not be hesitant to drop off a hoverboard in exchange for repairs at a company, but simply because you're a stranger who is on Craigslist and you could have repair clients who are hesitant to take the board.

Something to keep in mind with online shopping is that customers have six months to file charge-backs to their credit cards. When you buy items that are popular for high prices, there's a tendency for lots of fraud on credit cards. We'll address this in the next section.

Additionally, you should be worried about boards being broken by customers and then requesting a refund or charging back credit cards in the event that they are dissatisfied in the quality of the merchandise. In this regard, I would recommend paying slightly more for a high-quality product and avoid selling an inferior product, particularly when you accept PayPal, credit cards or any other way that allows charges back or disputes.

Additionally, you are able to sell locally. I use websites like Craigslist and Bookoo although there are million classified websites local to you.

Social media is also a an excellent place to sell. A few of my top re-sellers make much of their selling through social media websites such as Instagram, Facebook and Pinterest. There's also an abundance of classified apps online that you can download that you can download for your smartphone, including Offer Up Let Go, 5 Miles, and many more.

The advantage in selling local is that it's cash-based, so you do not have to worry about charges from credit cards or chargebacks.

Wholesaling

Wholesaling is the term used to describe selling to a different market, not just to the final consumer or retail customer and offering to businesses as well as sellers. Here's how it works.

I buy a pallet hoverboards, say 50 at an extremely low wholesale cost. I then look for other re-sellers willing to purchase boards from me and sell.

Instead of selling boards individually, I generally do not sell smaller then 10 boards one time. Ideally , I'm a middleman or broker deals with other brokers who are looking to purchase 50 boards at once.

I do not touch their products I simply accept their money and have board delivered to them directly and then I take the difference between the amount they pay me and the amount I will sell the boards to them. A bonus is that the more boards I offer the lower my prices get. Even if I'm only making marginal profits every order I receive as well as the greater business that I conduct can help me lower my own prices down.

A typical wholesale deal will look as follows. I will sell you a stack of boards for $250 per board. I purchase the boards from my supplier at a price of say $200 per board. I get $50 off each board purchased. If you purchase a pallet of 50 boards, I earned $50 off each one, which means I can earn $2500 in a single transaction and I do not need to handle the actual product. I buy it through my supplier and it is straight to the client at their house, in a warehouse or at a store.

The great thing about re-sellers is that they aren't as picky as buyers who are buying individually. For instance I sold a laptop to a woman for $400 in the week prior to the holiday. The night before Thanksgiving, she called me at 10:10 pm at night asking me to deliver her a new charger since she had broken hers.

One of my resellers would not bother me with questions such as this. They buy 50 boardsand when they encounter issues in one of them, of them, they will not blast my phone up or bother me. They'll simply return it the next time they purchase, and I'll exchange it to a brand new one for them, and then send the defective or damaged board back to the source to get the replacement.

Some wholesale deals are going to be made on complete pallets. I have sellers who visit three times per week and take five to 10 boards at one time. Your margins are likely to be lower when you buy wholesale because there is an amount of room for your sellers to earn a profit and since they buy in bulk, they can get better prices than a single. They are also moving more boards and you earn money by selling in bulk.

Apart from selling wholesaling boards I also have cellphone stores and electronics stores that sell my boards on consignment.

They don't need to raise any funds and I provide them with boards for free , but we share the profits on the boards they sell. Because they're part of a shop there's a little more trust from the perspective of potential buyers. They also have more value to be perceived and therefore, where I might be selling an item for $300 on Craigslist and they'll often have it for $500 at their shop.

I will charge them a little more on consignment boards since there's no risk for them and they're not required to pay any cash. This is a win-win situation for us and them. I make more money which is great for me. They earn an additional revenue stream from their business without needing to pay any money for boards.

When they're sold out, I stop by their store to settle what I owe them, and I offer them additional boards to market.

Parts

Parts is a relatively new sector. Hoverboards are damaged and require parts to fix them. There aren't many components inside the Hoverboard. There's the Shell frame, frames, two gyroscopes the motherboard, the battery and two wheels that include the motors for the wheels.

Parts are difficult to find and that's a good thing because it means that there aren't many vendors selling them. Parts aren't easy to locate is because hoverboards are so popular that manufacturers do not wish to sell their parts and instead utilize the components to make their own hoverboard and then market whole boards.

I began breaking down excellent boards into pieces boards, and I was surprised to discover I actually made more money by breaking up the board than make selling the entire board an excellent working board.

A hoverboard , for instance, cost me about $200. In that board, I've got two motors that I could sell in a set for up to $120 in an entire set or for $50. I have two motors that cost $150 to $100 for each wheel. I have a motherboard I can sell for $90 to $100 for.

Additionally, tiny parts such as the nipples, which transmit signals to the gyros cost $20 for a set, and it's just 2 pieces of rubber. If I split them out and then sell a complete board of components, I could occasionally get anywhere from $600 to $700, and I'm also able to get a working board for $450.

I've been able to locate some suppliers of parts and am now selling new factory parts , as an alternative to salvaged parts from boards, but it still is working. The margins on new items are very high as well. For instance, a gyroscope that I offer for sale at

$50, costs me just $6. The set of Nipples that I am able to sell for $17, will cost the buyer 0.60 cents. Sometimes, I make more profit on one piece as opposed to the entire board.

One thing I like about selling parts is that it's less hassle when selling the boards. In contrast, while Amazon has taken a hard line on selling Hoverboards and has required you to submit all kinds of documentation and receive approval, there aren't any rules or regulations on parts. Parts purchases are usually non-refundable, not just for hoverboards but with everything in general. This means that there is no need to worry about returns.

Repair

Repairing and repairing hoverboards has evolved into an extremely lucrative business. Hoverboards can be properly constructed, that is why they can are prone to breaking. Additionally, due to their nature even a well-constructed board could break if you use it for too long or use it in a way that is abusive.

The majority of people will need to fix them considering that they have paid hundreds of dollars for them. You can not only charge individuals for the component to repair their board but you could also complete your own repair and earn profits from the repair too.

The hoverboards don't really contain much. If something is wrong, it's basically going to have to be calibrated, to require the cables and connections checked or require just a handful of components. It's pretty easy to spot and correct issues when you take the time learning about these boards.

In reality, the majority of people doing repairs aren't experts or knowledge, they are taking a look at Youtube video clips or reading Reddit forums about how to fix their boards. Personally, I'm not very skilled, but I am able to repair almost any problem on the hoverboard.

This is how the repair game is played. Most often, you'll be charged for looking at the board regardless of whether you're able to repair your board or not. I charge $45, which means that even if I'm unable to repair your board, my time to examine it will cost you $45.

In terms of the actual repairs are concerned, you could charge for one repair, such as $80 for a replacement gyro however , due in the character of board you'll need to replace a few things or test different fixes before you can fix it.

The way some people go about it is to charge a flat repair price that is $185, regardless of the nature of the issue. Being a professional repairer, you'll always end up with the best outcome even if you need to replace or repair two gyros as well as the motherboard.

However, on the other hand there are times when you'll be lucky and the board might require just an initial calibration that takes of 30 seconds and you earn $185.

It could also be something more simple, like an inoperative wire that needs no components. If you need replacement for a gyroscope, for instance, you'll be in with a gyroscope that costs $6 and perhaps an hour of time. It's not bad for $185. Buyers also love it because they know that their board will be repaired and is expected to cost at least $185. Buyers aren't expecting any unexpected costs.

In terms of learning ways to repair these issues, it's as easy to watch Youtube videos and reading the hoverboard forums. If you encounter a problem that you're unable to fix it or find the answer, just join the SubReddit on hoverboards and ask for help, and someone will give you advice with suggestions on how to fix the issue.

Repairs to your hoverboard can be done on your own, either locally or through websites like Craigslist or create a website, and let customers send their boards to your company, and then make them pay for transportation of the board back to them when it's fixed and in addition to repairs and parts cost.

I also make an effort to contact other people within my region who are selling hoverboards, whether someone who has a warehouseor selling boards. Anyone who is going through 100-150 boards per week will have plenty of damaged ones. That's a huge amount of boards that you can fix. It's a benefit for them because instead of making a loss on a damaged board, they can have it repaired and then sell it to recoup the profits.

Chapter 4: Suppliers And Purchasing Your Inventory

If you decide to get into this field and have an online presence, you'll be able to be contacted by dozens of wholesalers, factories, and warehouses contacting and e-mailing them to offer you their products.

If you are just beginning, you'll be required to search for yourself some.

I started my journey with Ali Express buying a small amount of boards at each time. I quickly realized that the lengthy time to ship meant I was unable to meet the growing demand of boards. So I contacted Alibaba and began making contact with manufacturers in China.

I was able to purchase a vast quantity of boards at a reasonable price. Prices were excellent, but shipping via air was quite expensive. On an average, for 10 boards, I'd have to pay $900 for shipping. In most cases, shipping ended up costing twice as much as the boards. I bought the boards at a bargain but they still took a chunk of the profits.

Shipping by sea is possible that is very affordable, however it can take between 60-90 days to receive your package and you must manage all customs paperwork process yourself.

They will then be delivered to a port that is large, either Long Beach in California, Houston in Texas and New York. Then, it's your responsibility to determine how to deliver the boards at the ports. There are firms called freight forwarders that will take care of this on your behalf, with some cost of course.

I tried the Alibaba thing for a few months but I ended up finding wholesale boards in the US. I'd be willing to pay more, but the advantage is that the boards are available in the US with no wait.

A reliable wholesaler will also provide some assistance to you, too. If, for instance, I purchase a device that isn't working from the box, they will either return it and exchange it for a different one or at least , they will send me parts to repair it.

Another benefit for me was that I had to move lots of boards and could convince my supplier to include me to their insurance for product liability. Instead of paying between $2,000 and $3,000 to purchase my own product liability insurance since my wholesalers saw my ability to move their product and make me feel happy I was able to have my insurance covered for me.

Wholesalers are likely to be found within your locality but the largest ones with the highest rates are likely to be located near ports of California or Texas specifically with hoverboards. The majority seem to be directly from Long Beach in Cali or Houston in Texas.

A few things to be aware of when dealing with suppliers. If you buy through Ali Express it's easy and it's quite affordable, but remember that you're a retailer.

If you are ordering through Alibaba and you are a member of Alibaba, be aware that any less than a 100-piece order is considered to be a sample. This means that you're considered to be a non-priority for Alibaba. If an order that is large, 500 scooters is placed and your order is put on the lower end of the line until they are able to fill the order. It is not uncommon to be waiting over one month for your scooters to be manufactured and delivered.

In terms of the payment of your suppliers, never make payments via Western Union, there are plenty of frauds. Alibaba offers a variety of reliable methods. One is Ali Pay which is connected to Ali Express. The other one is known as T/T.

It's basically an Escrow system. When you wire a bank transfer to Alibaba but they don't release the funds for the manufacture until you receive the goods. This gives you additional protection for you.

Don't respond to emails sent by Chinese individuals from Alibaba that are not sent via Alibaba but rather to your personal email address. My experience is that it's usually employees of the factories that steal the contact information from their employers and attempt to make a profit to make money.

I have a friend who works in the field in China who has explained that salespeople only earn $500 per month. The factory workers earn even less. Many people try to earn an additional income by wooing US customers via email by using contact details from their work and then contact individuals by themselves. It is possible to send money using Western Union and will most likely never receive your product and you will never hear from them ever again.

My preference is USA sellers from the USA. Like I said, you are paying a bit more because a lot part of your work been completed for you, however you can avoid fraud. There is also more recourse in pursuing an individual who comes from the USA instead of China which has no chances of having your issue addressed.

Additionally, you don't need to worry about formalities for customs and the fees Additionally, you receive more support that can range from assistance with creating trucking companies to handle deliveries, as well as some help in the event of a bad products.

The people you buy from are purchasing tens or perhaps hundreds of thousands at each time from China They are important to factories and have more success in getting problems solved than if you bought some pallets on your own.

If I buy directly from US Warehouses, wholesalers or retailers, I usually pay between $190 and $250 based on the design of the board as well as whether it comes with Bluetooth or other options.

I could purchase $70 boards from China and after paying customs and shipping costs and the cost of freight forwarders, the cost is pretty similar to the price USA wholesalers sell to me for. However, I'd prefer to spend a little more and avoid the hassles, and a safer transaction.

If you are planning to do affiliate marketing, you're not going to be ordering physical items, so you won't have a supplier , so to say.

Most likely, you'll be selling on behalf of or as an affiliate for Amazon, eBay, Ali Express or an individual hoverboard seller's own website.

There's really nothing to discuss about this. Find out who's reliable and will actually pay affiliates. Personally, I believe eBay, Amazon, Ali Express are better over a random website for hoverboards which could disappear following the Holidays. Check out the affiliates' products pricing, costs, and commission rate to determine which is best suited to your requirements best.

In the final section, we'll discuss drop shippers and ways to locate a reliable provider for your drop shipping business. You can make use of something like Ali Express, however the delays in shipping could be a problem for certain customers, as the delivery times could be at the speed of two weeks, or the length of one month.

A few people prefer using Amazon as their drop-shipper. It is an option, but you'll need to need to do the best job at advertising your product and generating the value since Amazon can be a shopping site. Therefore, anyone who is looking to purchase from you can be able to easily take off your business and instead go to Amazon to look for other products.

The best option is to locate an agent or warehouse that can drop ship for you. I got a call from a man located in California who has more than 40000 pieces of inventory stored in his warehouse.

He could drop-ship boards to me at no cost for $216. This means that I can list the board on my own website or on eBay for $400. If it is successful in selling, I would pay him $216 and then he will deliver it to my customer. I manage the customer service aspects like collecting the cash and providing any support to the customer. If someone wishes to return the board, they must return it to my distributor in California.

Chapter 5: Liability Beware Of Scams And Losses

The product and the industry are more risky than other items sold on the internet. It is not only having to deal with the usual business concerns of finding trustworthy suppliers such as credit card charge-backs and fraud, and all that typical businesses have to face. Due because of the product's nature,, there are a variety of other aspects that you need to be aware of, for example, the possibility of someone suing you for hurting themselves on a board or because your board caused the house on the fire.

In this article, we'll look at the dangers of this business to avoid and the things to keep an eye on.

Liability

As I stated above that we live in a society that is litigious. If somebody falls off their board and is injured, they'll seek to blame. Somebody else than them. There are others seeking cash.

Typically, someone will to sue a company over the re-selling of a particular product, but you may be involved in the courtroom.

Not just over the accidents caused by the hoverboards as well as if one of your products catch on fire and burns a person's home down. This can be prevented by selling only high-quality products and instructing your customers about their use However, there's still some risk.

Although I'm not trying to scare the people around you, and I'm certainly not worried about being sued, but it's something you need to be aware of and consider the potential risks involved.

There are several ways to safeguard yourself. It is wise to establish an LLC or to incorporate.

If someone decides to sue you, they will only pursue the company not your personal assets or personal assets such as your home. It is not possible to sue you in a single instance, only your business is able to. It's something that everyone must take care of.

A thing to think about is purchasing product liability insurance, particularly when you are trying to build your own brand or expand your business. This usually is based off of the sales of your product, therefore when you're a new company you could have it fairly low since you'll be estimating your sales. It is possible to estimate on the lower range.

This will differ according to a myriad of factors, but after a thorough search for a million dollars in sales of hoverboards it is possible to pay between $2,000 and $3,000 for insurance on product liability.

I'm not saying that you should or shouldn't. Personally, I don't have any product liability insurance , though I'm incorporated and I think that gives me sufficient protection.

If I was privately labeling my hoverboards or trying to develop an own label, and was in the spotlight and trying to create an actual presence, I would purchase product liability insurance.

Scams

When making payments for items make sure you use the payment method that offers some level of transparency and recourse. A method such as Paypal, Ali Pay, or Alibaba T/T payment methods all come with some kind of buyer protection or an escrow.

A service similar to Western Union on the other on the other hand is nearly completely inaccessible and doesn't. While purchasing the samples of Chinese suppliers, I was cheated by Western Union for $500 three times in the course of sending money through Western Union.

There were other occasions when boards broke were delivered or I was cheated of boards when placing an order from China.

One time I tried Paypal that ended into covering my losses. in another instance, I was able to make an unauthorized charge to my credit card for one Ali Express purchase, and in another case, Ali Express buyer protection kicked into action and shielded me.

In most cases, when you receive damaged or defective boards due to the high shipping cost back to China the seller will try to reject a return or offer a refund in part of $30 or less. Some may even offer to send parts.

All well and great, but if aren't knowledgeable about how to repair boards, having it fixed professionally could end costing you much more than the service provider offers you. That is why having some kind of buyer protection beneficial.

Some other details about purchasing from China. It's not 100%, but I've experienced Chinese sellers tell methat If the seller is a person with an American name such as Jim Chan, don't deal with them. They're scammers. It's not 100 percent but it has saved me from scams several times.

Another tip is that before you deal with a vendor, check at their blacklist of suppliers. There is no guarantee that all bad sellers are on the list, but looking suppliers listed on the blacklist has stopped me from dealing with scammers in the past. It's something you must always do prior to engaging with any China supplier.

Finally, even for small samples, never transfer money via Western Union. There's no way to get a charge-back which leaves you vulnerable to fraud.

Theft from a Trucking Company

As I mentioned, it's more secure to purchase locally via USA Warehouses and wholesalers.

If you're not near them or are planning on picking the items yourself, you'll need to get it delivered to you. Contrary to smaller items, which can be delivered via USPS, UPS, FedEx or DHL Hoverboards are heavy and weigh around 25 pounds per piece, which means you'll have to hire an agency for trucking.

While UPS and FedEx offer an option for freight however, they are generally more expensive than using the trucking companies such as R&L as well as Roadrunner or any of the other.

When receiving truck shipments, always ensure that the pallet has an exact number of boards and not just "1 Pallet". If the pallet arrives but isn't full of boards, you don't have a recourse.

Demand that you are sure that the BOL or load bill, to state how many boards. If a trucking firm refuses to do this do not deal with them.

Typically, your USA supplier will usually be helpful and will have the knowledge to steer clear of scams and know how to handle it, making things much easier for you. My first load was a disaster although my supplier assisted me to in setting up for the load, it was my fault that I did not understand how to proceed and ended up losing two boards. I signed the load. It wasn't until I brought the load to my office that I realized that I was missing two boards. It was too for me to take action about the issue, however, since I already had signed the BOL that said that there fifty boards. I learned from the experience and from that point on, I always verified the number boards. If I saw a load with the words "pallet" in addition to the number of many boards it was, I would not accept the load.

Another thingto consider is to make sure the pallet you choose to use is evenly full cube. For instance, with standard 6.5" boards, typically pallets can hold 49 boards. This is 7 rows of seven boards.

A lot of suppliers want to ship 50 since it's an even number. If you send 50 boards, each time you'll only get one board. The reason is because the cube is equal with one board that is loose covered with plastic wrap.

In the course of time, an employee from the warehouse or a trucking employee may cut the plastic and take the loose board , if they are aware of what's inside the pallet

You've probably heard of the phrase, "it fell off the back of an automobile" when it comes to the theft of merchandise. There's a reason why that phrase is in use, since there's plenty of thefts from trucking and warehouses.

Another thing to look out for is. Your cargo is covered, but generally, you will be charged an deductible of $500. Trucking employees are aware of the possibility of stealing two boards from you and you won't have to file any claim since the claim could cost more than the two boards stolen. The amount of the claim is $500, and two boards would cost $400-$450.

You can guard yourself against theft by taking several steps.

Make sure you choose a reputable trucking firm. Third, only ship full pallets made up of 49 pieces or any other size that makes one an equal cube. This may differ in eight" or 10-" boards since the boxes differ in size. Thirdly, always verify each pallet and weigh it. if you're not satisfied, don't sign the BOL for the entire load. Keep track of how many pieces you got and share it with your trucking firm and your supplier at a later time.

Finally, you should make sure that your wholesaler shipping your boards to take two steps. The first is to make use of the black plastic wrap rather than clear, so nobody can tell what's in the pallet. It could be a brands like raisin instead of expensive hoverboards that nobody knows about.

Additionally, they produce tapes that are tamperproof. It is taped prior to when it's sent out and in the event that you open the box, altered with, or repacked , you can tell.

Broken Boards

Broken boards will be the most costly loss. When you're having to deal with many boards, it is likely that there will be some faulty boards or damaged from shipping.

This is the reason it's crucial to talk to your supplier about the kind of assistance they can provide. Are they willing to return boards that have been damaged? If they don't want to accept them back, can they provide with spare parts for fixing them on your own or pay for someone else to repair them?

You will also have either retail customers or clients who are reselling your products likely to claim that the boards are damaged.

Before you sell, you must decide on your policy is. Are all sales final for the customers are entirely on their own? Are you willing to give them a 24-hour window to check out and return boards, as in the event of no physical harm?

Plan out how you will go to deal with your customers Create an policy, clearly communicate the policy to your customers, and follow it.

Something I've done several times that I have been successful in is to provide two prices for my wholesalers.

You can, for instance, purchase boards for $280 each and receive support, parts or replacements. You can also purchase boards for $225, but you're completely on your own.

At $280, I'm earning enough money to eat some boards , and offer some parts for free. At $225 , my margins are so low that eating one board can make me lose the profits of the sale of 10-12 boards.

The majority of my customers choose to buy at a lower cost but if they experience an issue , I inform them to be patient. I'll either replace their damaged boards for the lowest price, and then they will pay the difference or fix the boards for them, for the cost of.

I'm not even going to look at boards that costs less than $25, and should I need to perform an repair, I charge them for labor and parts. It's a risk they make on their own on whether they'd prefer an affordable cost and hope that everything goes as planned, or if they'd prefer to pay more and get assistance.

A damaged or broken board are likely to be the biggest loss for you, so be sure to have a plan in place with your suppliers and your clients.

Credit Card Charge-backs and Returns

This is only true for those who sell online or for those who decide to use debit cards at the counter. Hoverboards can be a costly product, so you'll make more sales if you purchase credit cards instead of cash. However, it exposes you to charge-backs on credit cards because of fraud or unhappy customers.

I'll be sharing an interesting background with you. Soldier Boy the rapper came out with his own hoverboard that he named "the Soldier Board.

He created the Shopify store that accepted Shopify payments using Stripe. The store was able to pay $250,000 fraudulent charge-backs to credit cards. He was featured in the media crying over this, and asking why Shopify didn't Shopify stop the chargebacks.

Shopify actually has fairly good fraud detection features, however it's important to actually keep an eye on the filters.

Soldier Boy had not logged into his account for more than six weeks. He was believed to have another person working for him , namely monitoring orders and packing and shipping them.

It was not until the charge-backs were issued that it was clear that he'd made all of these orders that were fraudulent.

It's a bit of a pity of his own, however it's something that you need to be vigilant about. You can guard yourself by limiting your shipping to a credit card's billing address. This can dissuade some buyers, however you could also request a photo of the back and front of the card as well as an ID.

Another seller ioHawk is currently in debt to Shopify Payments over $900,000 or more than a million dollars in charge-backs resulting from fraudulent charges. I'd think that a larger company that has a more knowledgeable businessperson, like Tony Hawk, would avoid similar situations, however, these two cases illustrate the severity of the issue.

Alongside plain fraudulent purchases Many sellers on the internet don't know that customers can avail a credit card bareback up to 6 months following the purchase.

If you offer a board to someone but it breaks two months later and you decide not to fix it, they could be able to file an action against their card provider in order to receive their money back. Then you're owed this money to the merchant processor.

If you intend to use cards, ensure you charge sufficient for the boards that your margins will allow the possibility of reimbursements, or even replacement boards.

In the example above, if you're only making $20 per board each board you sell will wipe out 10 sales on a board if your costs per board are $200.

On the other hand, if you sell boards for $600 and then you return an item, you could easily afford sending 3 replacement boards to customers and remain profitable and in the black.

Last point I'll discuss as a method to sell on the internet and stay clear of charge-backs.

A new service is available named "Pay Near Me". What it does is that you make a purchase by you on the internet. You give them the QR code which they can print or display on their mobile.

The customer can then take the number to any 711 location, CVS and Dollar Store and pay in cash. There are no charge-backs and the money is completely cleared and available for withdrawal within 3 days.

It is a secure way to sell on the internet, offering an easy payment option however, it's not as easy as credit cards, and you can avoid credit card fraud or charge-backs in the future.

Chapter 6: What To Sell

In this section , I'll explain to you the best way to promote and market you Hoverboard Self Balance Scooters.

I'm not going into the details of the various ways to market and promote sales since that would be a whole book. If you're looking for, check out my other books and programs that will teach you in-depth on affiliate marketing and guerrilla marketing video marketing, etc.

In this article, we'll discuss the best ways to market and sell based on whether you're an affiliate marketer drop shipper, wholesaler or retailer. It also depends on whether you're planning to sell locally or online, too.

Wholesaler

Wholesalers are seeking wholesalers who are re-sellers. That means you're not looking for the final buyer, but only those who are reselling.

Here's how I locate my sellers who are re-sellers. I visited flea markets in my area and approached sellers selling electronic gadgets, airsoft guns or any other item whose intended audience is hoverboards. I tried selling to them.

I stumbled across some vendors at flea markets selling hoverboards. I contacted them and informed me I was able to beat price. This is how I snagged several sellers.

The Offer-Up, Craigslist, Bookoo and other local classifieds performed well as well. Not only did I include in my ads for retail however, I also offered wholesale. If I saw any other businesses who had high costs or low quality boards, I would call them and ask to become their wholesaler. This allowed me to get many wholesale accounts.

I also visited local electronics stores and repair shops for cell phones. I also sold boards to some while others made consignment agreements with me.

The way a consignment deal operates is that I'm basically the money-maker. I purchase the boards and they put them into their shop. They don't charge a cent. They are selling 10 boards. When they're gone, I pay my cash and donate them another 10.

Usually, I am able to charge them more than those who purchase their own merchandise since it creates a revenue stream for their business without having to spend any cash or take on any risk.

Cellphone stores and even small electronic shops that sell drones as well as other gadgets are the most recommended places to visit and head shops.

In addition, I utilized Social Media, Youtube, as well as the usual methods you'd use to promote any business to get wholesale customers. A final thing to add. Do not limit yourself to only your local area.

I would like to place ads across all cities as and also contact customers from every city. Since boards can be transported via truck, you don't have restrict yourself to your geographical location.

One obstacle to overcome is that people aren't confident sending $10,000 to someone else with the assurance that boards will be delivered by truck three days later. But when you're professional it is possible to do so.

Drop Shipping and Retail

We've covered a lot on selling these products through retail. If you're interested in going on eBay or Amazon or even your

own Shopify website. If you prefer to deal with local Craigslist, Bookoo, Flea Markets.
As I mentioned above Social Media sites like Youtube, Facebook and Instagram are excellent places to display your product and attract potential buyers.

You may be stocking inventory or dropping shipping the methods to bring traffic to your store online are basically the same. Pay-per-click advertising, blogs and videos on the internet that include links to your shop.
I'm a big advocate of two platforms that are free such as Blogger and Youtube for making reviews, unboxing and review videos and repair videos that increase traffic.
Give the reader with value. For instance, someone who wants to purchase a hoverboard probably search for reviews. Write a review that includes the link to your product . And when someone views the review and is impressed by the product, there is a high chance they'll buy.
Repair videos are particularly useful in selling parts. When you've got a video that will not just identify someone's issue for them and then show the steps to resolve it

as well as the item to sell it is an excellent method of driving sales for parts.

This time, I'll not talk about specifically Affiliate Marketing as the same strategies used to bring customers to your online shop are also able to be employed to bring customers to your affiliate's store.

Another thing I'll suggest is to take on "long Tail Keywords". If you're marketing something similar to Hoverboards on the internet, you must to be ranked in Google and appear on search results for keywords similar to Hoverboards.

Hoverboards can be used to connect all sorts of items. You want to convince buyers to click, so you need to add "long Tail Keywords" A buyer might be looking for just prior to hitting the trigger and making the purchase.

A few Examples of Long Tail Keywords could include...

"Which hoverboard should I purchase?"

"Which hoverboard comes with an extended warranty?"

"What is the highest high-quality hoverboard?"

These kinds of phrases will be the last thing someone is looking for prior to making a purchase. That is why you need to keep them on the buying journey just before they pull the trigger and use the credit card.

Distinguishing Yourself From The Competition

There are many people selling Hoverboards in the local market and on the internet. What can you do to differentiate yourself from the crowd?

I enjoy making infographics with side-by-side contrasts of my boards against the boards of competitors. It could be the material used, the method by which they are constructed, the quality of battery that is used in them, etc. I emphasize the unique features and components on my board that differentiate them than others and include the boards in marketing material. Below provides an illustration of what I'd make.

=

Some of the more frequent customer queries will be, what kind of battery the board is equipped with? What's the name of the manufacturer? Does it have a guarantee?

For brands, they mean something to consumers, but in reality, they do not refer to quality. It's the Razor Scooter hoverboard, which costs approximately three times as costly than most boards is not as well-reviewed as other boards. Customers do like to know about brands, in just like the majority of customers purchase Fruity Pebbles over the generic Fruity Corn Cereal.

I was connected to an online retailer who had already supplied an branded board and box. Even if you're getting generic boards , it's fairly simple to design an own branding.

You can purchase your own box and packaging designed for inexpensive, perhaps less than $4 for a box. On the other hand, you can hire someone to design your own letters or logos on vinyl to apply and print on the board.

You're is selling the same basic boards that 100 other companies are, but you can name you're The Fly Board or any other clever name you'd like to think of. Below are some images of a custom-designed box against a generic one.

For batteries, everybody seems to get stuck about Samsung as well as LG batteries.

Many are Chinese batteries that have counterfeit stickers. I've seen several companies confirm to me that they are Chinese batteries, and then slap an Samsung or LG sticker on the battery.

One thing you need to be aware of is that neither Samsung neither LG produce genuine hoverboard batteries. They manufacture battery cells that can be combined with a computer board in order to create a hoverboard-style battery, but they don't make hoverboard batteries.

It isn't possible to tell whether you've got an Samsung or LG battery until you take the battery apart and look at the cells or even then, it might be fake cells.

If you can get the best battery available, there's no reason to spend more or be hung up about purchasing the best Samsung as well as an LG battery.

In the end, warranty is something that everyone would like to have. I was a bit surprised even selling on Craigslist to find that numerous buyers inquire about the warranty.

To the extent that they are not applicable, warranties are essentially useless. If you purchase from China they will provide you with an one-year warranty but you're responsible for shipping both to and from China, which means you are getting between $250 and $300 in shipping costs that is more than the cost of purchasing a new board.

A few USA sellers provide a warranty but they usually offer their boards for $600 or more, which basically means that the buyer is purchasing a second board in advance. Sellers are more than tripled their profits in the sale, therefore if they need to send a second replacement board, so be it.

Finally, some sellers provide you with the option to purchase a warranty between $150 and $300.

Like all warranties, they usually only cover specific parts for example, with hoverboards typically batteries and motherboards. They do not cover abuse or misuse, therefore, as with all warranties, purchasers will likely be informed that they are not covered or they misused the product, and may end out not being covered by the warranty.

If you're planning to offer a guarantee, that is your choice, however I would suggest to ensure that you are earning at least two times your profit on a single board, or even three times the amount so that you are able to afford repairs or replace a piece of equipment without having to cut into your profits. Also, be certain of the terms of the warranty, what it covers and doesn't cover, who pays shipping costs, and any other details that your customer might disagree with you regarding.

Chapter 7: The Hoverboard Manual

You can find a hoverboard equipped with ABS plastic shells, ABS is a form of plastic made from which

It is extremely tough and robust, it won't break or split on collision,

It can take many knocks and won't fall apart. A lot of hoverboard shells

They are made of PVC made of PVC. PVC plastic is prone to cracking and break, and it is also

get weaker and more vulnerable after being exposed to sunlight.

A hoverboard isn't going to last five minutes with this kind of plastic. Some hoverboards

They are made from stainless steel. This results in them being more expensive.

Believe it or not, they are not as durable in terms of endurance and elimination of

Dents and bumps are ABS plastic. The stainless steel forms an

indentation or distortion when it is hit it, resembling an accident in a car!

2. You pay for what you get for

Find a hoverboard that costs $390.00 or more, the cheapest

Versions with lower quality wheels as well as axles, shells and electronics , and the overall

Manufacturers will make cuts throughout the entire process to cut costs. You can do it yourself

A balance scooter must be a mix of premium design and cutting-edge

magic, don't do it to save $100, it's a scam and you'll end up spending about

If you spend more than $390, your life will be better for it. like many other things in life, you'll get what you pay for.

You are paying you pay.

3. Insider secrets - PCB

In the less expensive hoverboards they also come with the circuit that is of low quality

board, also known as "PCB" PCB is made up of all the microelectronics as well as silicon chips.

run your board effectively The less expensive versions will not last as long, and they aren't

constructed from low-quality electrical circuitry which contain non-standard chips as well as low-quality.

high-quality wiring and fuses Beware of that scam and purchase the versions that don't have the quality.

They are usually priced between $280 and $300.

4. Purchase from Amazon or another reputable retailer

Shop on Amazon or from a trusted supplier All Amazon suppliers must

are subjected to strict tests of quality and performance and must be able to maintain

particular standards regarding timely delivery cancellation, customer service and timely shipping orders.

On a regular basis on a daily basis. You can also read reviews from customers and check out what others have said about them.

The public is thinking, so you can find out the facts on what the hoverboard

Are you thinking of purchasing. Be careful before buying on Ebay or any other website, Does the seller has a return policy? What is the part warranty? What are the conditions of the warranty?

numerous positive reviews are there?

5. Do not be concerned over Chinese imports!

It's hard to believe however, the hoverboard was developed and was first licensed in
China is not Germany and neither is the USA China, not Germany or the USA! There are hoverboards from the USA and Europe. European and US hoverboards

Manufacturers would like you to believe they have a $800-1200 hoverboard is the best.
authentic article, while authentic product, and Chinese versions are counterfeits, but not
true! True! Chinese invented the invention in 2014, and have continued to do so ever since. they
They have licensed the patent to a variety of Chinese companies, mostly based in
the high-tech manufacturing in Shenzhen China near Hong Kong. The US as well as European manufacturers are trying to charge a higher price for their products.
The same applies to you, don't let yourself be taken advantage of or fooled by false impressions of quality.

7 reasons that self-balancing scooters will be here to stay , and not just
A trend
1. They're great fun!
The thrill never fades when you have a self-balancing scooter or hoverboard. they
They are so enjoyable to usethat you get the feeling of riding on a wave of air when you creatively pirouette and dance through town. It's an easy task to
It takes just 10 minutes to master, you'll never regret feeling this liberated
and simple. The hoverboard is a great way to lift your spirits and send you on the right track to
an exciting beginning to your day.
2. There are so many places to visit
If you don't live in the Rockie mountains or on the gentle mountain slopes Mount Everest,
You have millions of locations you can go using your own.
scooter, all hoverboards of good quality will withstand an upward steep slope of 20 degrees
The incline of nearly every walkway, shopping centre and open-air park has an

You are yours to go for a spin, jump onto your hoverboard and go out and about.
Explore the world.
3. Eliminates the energy from long-distances and produces zero emissions
Are you thinking of visiting Starbucks in your neighborhood? Starbucks? Perhaps you're running behind to get there?
Your appointment with a chiropractor to you heal your hip pain? Don't worry,
Forget about the pedals or car With the hoverboard, you can go anywhere
Much faster than walking, and you can also use the paths and sidewalks to gain speed.
to get there, and in addition, the hoverboard is all you need
charging overnight and ready to use the entire day long. There is no need to charge overnight.
pollutants like your car, and has no mechanical energy as on your bike It's
A win-win for both you and the earth!
4. They're cheap to manage
Parking and petrol bill for car mechanics and oil changes, operating an
The automobile of today is expensive, and in certain countries, there is tax

Also, you can pay by using your self-balancing scooter, you are able to avoid all of these
fees and only use nighttime electricity to power your scooter
batteries. You can purchase a carrying case for $20-25 and then use the
It's easy to carry around since it weighs only 10 kilograms You'll have no excuses.
You can save money while having the time of your life!
5. It's easy to stay clear of congestion and reach locations promptly
Do not be worried about being late for an appointment or yoga class or your yoga
or even meeting your next employer or meeting your next employer, just or ride the hoverboard

footplates on the outside of your front door and racing! Avoid rush hour
travel and don't forget an important date. use your umbrella when you believe it's
it's likely to rain and you'll appreciate the ride better than the snarling of
Trap-like traffic, with angry drivers, carbon monoxide leaking out.

turning into smog. A self-balancing scooter gives you lots of freedom, and also
There is no test for driving you have to pass!
6. It's got plenty of social evidence!
Do you believe in the hype?? We disagree, with over 2 million self-balancing
scooters were sold all over the world during the six months leading up until June 2015, and the they are in high demand.
is growing so fast, certain companies have even sold their entire
stock for Christmas, but we don't have this amazing method of transportation
is likely to go out of business in the near future is not likely to happen anytime soon, so get your self-balancing scooter today.
today!
7. They're equipped with a variety of technology and are easy to keep clean
You can also buy the hoverboard, which comes with Bluetooth and speakers
Nowadays, you can simply power up your smartphone's music collection and
Get it in the streets! It's a good idea to be more conscious of what you are doing in the social world.

Other than this .... So you can listen in silence on your Bluetooth headphones or Wireless headsets instead. Additionally, newer models come with a wireless headset.
wireless technology as well as remote control handsets, and, in the near future, we could witness
Google Glass with integrated Google-glass functionality as well as collision avoidance systems that integrate google-glass functionality and collision avoidance.

Five Fun Things to Do on your hoverboard
If you're hoping to get the most of enjoyment from your
If you're a hoverboard user, explore these five bizarre activities:
1. Bring your pet out for a stroll along the wild side
A lot of parks have gently flowing walkways as well as gravel paths. are
A hoverboard is easy to ride on. Go out into the wilderness and take in the beautiful countryside.

The natural world, including nature and greenery can be beneficial for mental well-being, and has been proven

Scientifically proven that 15 minutes of exposure to greenery for 3 times every week is scientifically proven that 15 minutes exposure to greenery over 3 times per

could lead to the reduction of stress in more than 95% of adults.

For more entertainment, you can put your dog's favorite pet on a lead and go for a walk

Also, get one of those stretch leads because you don't want to be in a serious accident to happen.

When your dog sees an animal and then zooms off to the side, while you're standing still

On top of your bike.

2. Form your own biker gang and link arms!

Have always wanted to join The Hells Angels but couldn't afford an Harley Davison? Do it! to get a lower-cost alternative, you and your companions purchasing selffor less.

using balance scooters and placing yourself in a continuous human chain

With your shoulders and hands, you can create an e-hoverboard train. You will not only get a lot done, but you will also
of your friends, you don't have to endure the hells of Hells Angels initiation
It's like riding in full speed against an unfinished brick wall, or getting inks that aren't so good.
3. Try it using the help of a handstand
Safety Alert! We do not recommend this to the typical Joe but only if
You're a gymnast, or acrobat. However, you're also the movement is forward and moving your hands in a backward direction while holding your hands, could be among the most stunning
Hoverboard tricks we've seen.
4. Go for it in the skateboard park
Are you looking to reconnect with your lost youth or relax on the skateboard
Chicks and dudes? Go to your local skateboard park , which is perfect for both.
The ideal way to test your agility, balance and ability to balance, but be cautious
Be careful not to leap on and off your hoverboard using lots of force to force

yourself onto or off your hoverboard. They aren't
built to handle large loads or forces, or even break into two!
5. You can drive through rush hour traffic with the most smug smile at your face!

Five things you should not do on your hoverboard
1. Get on board! Hoverboards are not made to handle huge forces or force,
They'll crack under the strain and stress So don't even attempt it.
2. Take two people on your hoverboard will be able to take control 40-150 kilos if you are careful.
However, this tends to be one person only made, and you're
taking a small safety risk since balancing is difficult with two people
3. Let it fall into the water. Many hoverboards have splash protection or
Showerproof, then put in the pool and the game is done!
4. Modify it - there are many YouTube videos that show how to modify it.

Modify it to fit larger kerbs with less difficulty However, any modifications made could be a problem.

It can invalidate the warranty provided by the manufacturer It will invalidate the warranty, so don't do it!

5. You can charge it. The lithium-ion battery within your hoverboard requires

charging, and if you keep it on charge, after it has run out of battery,

If you do, you'll be limiting the life of your battery, so charge it as much as you can in between

is used to extend battery life. New batteries cost around $50 however, which is a great deal

It's not the end of the world if you require an upgrade within 3-4 years.

Five fantastic safety tips to keep in mind for your hoverboard

1. Always wear a safety helmet be safe always wear a head protection as

you don't even know what happens when a random person accidently knock you down.

If you fall off and hit you head against the pavement, avoid taking the chance to take the risk.

Put on a safety headgear.

2. Use elbow and knee padsto prevent cuts and bruises , as well as dislocated

kneecaps and elbow joints. imagine yourself as an urban skateboarder,

A set of elbow and knee pads may cost less than $20.

3. Do not swerve into and out of people - do not be an antisocial liar,

weaving between and around pedestrians is reckless and dangerous It could be dangerous, and it can cause injury.

Feel like you're having a blast however, it's also the quickest way to cause an accident. You could

can seriously hurt someone else that you weren't planning to do.

4. Don't attempt jumpsas your hoverboard might snap and break in the blink of an eye.

when you apply a significant amount of force on it try to avoid by jumping over it

5. Don't drive on the roadsand stay off the highways or roads It's first filled with

vehicles that are fast-moving that could hit you, and then you may be struck by
be arrested since it is not motor vehicle.

Self-Balancing Scooters are worth the price? money?-
Skateboarding, Segway's and scooting have become a regular part of our lives.
Modern technology makes getting around a bit more enjoyable. The latest kid on the block.
The blocks is the Self-balancing Scooter, or The Hover Board. There are a lot of
Coming to market, But which of them is best for you? I've done some research
about them and which one on them is the best. Check out the following article to discover what I've discovered.
What is the Self-balancing Scooter?
The Self-Balancing scooter can be described as an electric motor that has two wheels powered miniature Segway. It's
The driver's movement is the sole control controlled by the driver's movement, similar to how controlled by the driver's movements, similar to how a Segway is controlled by the driver's movement. Lean

forward, and your electronic motor comes to move you forward, leaning
From side to side to move the Self-Balancing scooter in the direction of objects, or away from them.
the road. The road has been receiving a lot of media attention from Celebrities like Justin
Bieber, Chris Brown and Cesc Fabregas are all involved and joining in the action along
Their personal self-balancing scooters. You can find them their Instagrams and
YouTube what amount can be awaited on one.
The Self-Balancing Scooter is equipped with the following features:
Durable Tyre's-
All models come with rubber tires that are durable to ensure that they are able to
take care of the bumps and uneven surfaces they encounter on the surface of the sidewalk.
Fully equipped with Over-Tyre guards that stop any debris from flying over the user's head.

pants or clothes. They also allow an excellent product that will last for many years. the item

They are designed to ensure that nails and stones don't cause problems for them.

Speed-

Typically, these products fall in the range of 6-10MPH , based on the

The model of the company you buy. It has just the perfect amount of speed for your

Your excitement levels are at a high level, but you are safe and kept.

which makes it the best choice in terms of speed.

Agility-

Because of the low-profile design of the self-balancing scooter, it can be an attractive

A smooth and agile ride that is designed to be fast and easy to get in and from turns just like an experienced professional

Skier, it fulfills all of its goals. There are a few determining elements that determine which

Scooter is likely to become the fastest, however it all is largely due to the size of the wheel.

and the scooters length, and The scooters Length, 1.1m tall, 35cms long

and 50cms wide. Anything larger than that becomes a than a sluggish and a more sluggish ride and 50cms wide. Anything larger than this becomes a more lull user.

Design-

There are two main designs that are a part of the forward runners of the self-balancing Scooter. They're a circular version versus the more angular

squarer products. For me , the more circular-shaped product wins in

The test of design to see how they perform, and this is the reason. The Circular designed Self-balance scooter has passed

It is more sleek and slimmer in comparison to the more angular model. It is also less bulky and more streamlined.

It is lighter and more easy to maneuver when you're out slightly lighter and easier to maneuver when users are. The other

A cool and unique feature is very cool feature of the front-facing L.E.D's that light up when the user is taking the board taking on the board, taking the board, L.E.D lights are more to offer than just an attractive accessory

purpose, and by using the feature of having the L.E.D's located at the top side of the Scooter it enhances the appearance of the Scooter.

it is very easy for pedestrians to be able to see the pedestrian as they come down the

pavement, particularly at night . It is also crucial to keep in mind that you should not walk on

This is not intended for use on roads the sidewalk is right close to

the roadway and the lights assist in making sure the drivers know users on the road. The lights and roadside help ensure that drivers are aware of users on

Side of the side of the.

Chapter 8: Advantages And Use Of Self-Balancing Electronic Scooters And Electronic Hoverboards

Invading technologies, technologies that have a profound impact on
traditional techniques and established markets are always welcomed with enthusiasm.
scepticism. But, as with the introduction of automobiles to replace horses
and carts, and the use with computers to provide a substitute for pen and
pencil, their existence challenges the existing technology and ultimately proves to be
an effective replacement, or at the very least, a viable alternative with benefits
typically, they far surpass their predecessors or market leaders.
Self-balancing scooters are the most advanced examples of this technology.
Despite initial ridicule and discrimination however, their benefits and use have been proven
be wide-ranging and continually growing.

Electronic transport is growing more widespread,
Fashionable fashion with Segway sales increasing by 25%, as well as the latest generation of self-balancing
scooter is set to make huge advancements in the market.
This is not just a marketing gimmick for those who are fashion-conscious, but an array of industries and segments
They are using them as part of their daily practice. It is easy to switch from
from indoors to outside everything is available from the emergency department to campus of the university
and music festivals are utilizing and benefiting from hoverboards
technology and the incorporation of self-balancing scooters is new and exciting technology.
the market is constantly growing and shareholders are showing no signs of slowing.
Here's a list of their many benefits as well as examples of their comprehensive
reach.
Eco friendly

Self-balancing scooters are powered by lithium-ion batteries, and therefore are by nature
zero-emission devices that operate both inside and out and thus
increasing their useability. With companies, governments and people being
Pressure to reduce the carbon footprint of electronic transportation is fast becoming a way to reduce their carbon footprint.
increasing in popularity and a green alternative to the conventional.

Cost effective
The cost of fuel and car maintenance cost continue to rise, putting pressure on the electronic
scooter is a popular alternative mode of transport. The cost of
technology for hoverboards and scooters, and maintenance is also decreasing , which
In turn, they are reducing their prices to customers while the same can't be said about
the auto industry and its related costs.

They ease the job
In the following various industries are using self-balancing scooters

in order to boost productivity and decrease the amount of energy expended by humans and the amount of time
consumption. All from law enforcement officers to gas meters inspectors
and delivery personnel are utilizing the advantages of electronic hoverboards as well as
Integrating into their day-to-day operations. They have access to areas that other vehicles aren't able to.
Microchip Technology's Portland base makes use of electronic transportation to transport its two
Double benefit of the reduction of human effort and workload and ensuring the purity and hygiene. The freeway that connects them is built to allow for self-balancing
scooters to transport people and resources without contamination of their
campus.
Security and medical treatment

Not only do law enforcement personnel utilize self-balancing scooters, but also security during live events and festivals are now using them. The new technology is now being used

The vantage point offers an additional advantage in field of view and speed

The hoverboards' design allows them to respond quickly and effectively.

In Chicago there is a two-person paramedic team patrols the city . They can provide treatment

rapid emergency assistance as seen the scene in Salt Lake City where

Electronic boards are utilized to gain access to the areas that are congested and not accessible by

vehicle.

Interestingly, self-balancing scooters are being put to good use in

teams of bomb disposal around the world, fully loaded with bomb disposal equipment.

professionals able to maneuver their additional 120 pounds worth of safety equipment

with ease, and bomb disposal specialists able to conserve their energy

and concentration to carry out and focus for.

As the price of gas continues to increase, so does environmental responsibility, and the associated
cost continue to rise and as ever more government agencies, industries and
people are exploring the possibility of self-balancing scooters, the usage of personal
Electronic transportation is set to increase in the coming years and also disrupt
The status quo can be maintained with their possibilities limit only by the size of
the human brains operating their minds.
These are the Top 10 Cities In Which You Can Ride Your Hoverboard
So, you've got your self-balancing board, and you're surrounded by new
potentialities waiting for you to discover. What are you waiting for? Where do you go with advantage of it?
Its incredible range of capabilities? With the hoverboard , you can reinvent your experience
Enjoy the city in all its glory experience, and taking in all the sights and attractions from a singular and innovative

new perspective. Here's a list of some of the most beautiful destinations in the world.
Take the new bike you bought.

1. Prague

The city is known as "the City of a Hundred Spires," Prague is famous for its vibrant Baroque structures, Gothic churches, medieval Astronomical Clock, and beautiful women.

The view is from Old Town Square, Charles Bridge, Wenceslas Square and Prague Castle the

The architecture of this city is breathtaking. The use of electronic transportation is so widespread in this city that the local authorities recently declared war against Segway use. That's quite a bit.

Demand and the nature-based beauty Prague is an absolute must for everyone hoverboard adventurers.

2. London

London is a modern city in the 21st century, however with a rich history dating back to Roman times. With such a huge space of wonders of the world to discover there

There is perhaps no better place for a self-balancing scooter than London. Make the Thames be your
guide to help you enjoy the stunning sights from Big Ben, Westminster Abbey and the Houses of
Parliament or go to The Olympic Village and the sporting venues that are scattered throughout the
city.

3: Los Angeles

Fly through Angel City while taking to the sights of the world's
Entertainment capital. It is located in to the Hollywood Hills, Santa Monica Boulevard and
Venice beach, from the tours from Warner Brothers and Paramount Studios you'll be
you'll likely meet one of the celebs of the A-list hoverboard enthusiasts on your way.

4. Barcelona

One of Europe's most amazing cities that has vast expanses of coastline line to discover along
with its labyrinth-like character of the city's centre, in which the streets appear to develop

and change with the seasons and you'll never get bored exploring the highest peaks of
The Camp Nou and the pleasure of the golden beach. With streets that change to
Sand, Barcelona is truly one of Europe's most beautiful cities. It is should be on your list of destinations.
self-balancing scooter adventure.

5: San Francisco
San Francisco is the home to a bit of everything. Maximise the beauty of
Enjoy this amazing city without the strain of climbing hills. Enjoy the sights of
Views and practice your self-balancing skills, with unbeatable access to the
Bay, Golden Gate Bridge, Alcatraz and Fisherman's Wharf. Try your hand at a variety of challenges while you
take a stroll along the streets of fame.

6: Munich
The most unique cities and possibly Germany's most appealing,
Enjoy the Bavarian culture and soak up the stunning surroundings. It's where you can call home.

of Oktoberfest But don't get caught up in the local food or
The task of balancing your hoverboard could be difficult while you explore Marienplatz as well as and Gothic Neues Rathaus.

7: Rome

In Rome Modern and ancient and past, present and future exist in the same place. Make sure you are aware
A balance scooter that is balancing in an exciting journey through one of the most well-known and renowned
historic cities, exploring all the attractions including The Colosseum up to the Pantheon and
Vatican City.

8: Amsterdam

The most bike-friendly city is home to a vibrant and innovative art scene
World-renowned museum and more than 165 canals for you to discover. With hundreds of kilometers
of cycling paths, of cycle paths. This is the ideal city to explore using your hoverboard. The city

The most famous tourist attractions offer everything for everyone, starting with the Anne Frank house to Anne Frank house
from Dam Square this city if the future of transportation is electronic.

9: Sentosa

One of Asia's most sought-after tourist destinations, favored by more than 20 million people.

annual population of a million, Sentosa has 2km of protected beaches, and areas of exceptional

natural beauty as well as golf courses and hotels and the stunning Merlion statue

Singapore's national symbol and the national symbol. An immense expanse of land to be

Explored and tested your hoverboarding abilities.

10: Dubai

Famous for its modern designs, luxury shopping, and a lively nightlife

Dubai is a world-class destination with world-class attractions. the skyline is dotted with towering skyscrapers

eagerly waiting to navigate with fashion. Perhaps there is no place better than the

perfect location for a hoverboard than the city of New York.
A new era than this futuristic city that features controlled lighting
You can practice to improve your self-balancing skills.

UNCATEGORIZED
Which stars are fans of self-balancing scooters?
What are Justin Bieber, Chris Brown, Nick Jonas, Zedd, Soulja Boy, Kendall Jenner,
JR Smith, Nicki Minaj, Wiz Khalifa, Karim Benzema as well as Skrillex all have their own in
common? They love self-balancing scooters.
The Hollywood Hills, shopping malls, kitchens and bedrooms , to aeroplanes
and and the Las Vegas strip, it's impossible to escape the excitement of these groundbreaking
New hoverboards are taking the world of celebrity by storm and are quickly becoming a household name.
A vital element that is a part of pop culture.
Twitter, Instagram YouTube, Facebook and Twitter are all

of celebrities raving about these devices that are game-changing and the entire of the comments of celebrities raving about these devices. All of the comments
asking two simple questions: what is it and how do I get it? !
Here's a list with the most popular fans in the world of celebrities along with what's been doing.
and.
Jamie Foxx:
Hollywood major-hitter Jamie Foxx introduced the world to self-balancing
scooter as he rode on his scooter to Tonight Show with Jimmy Fallon. The first
Ambassadors set the ball rolling, and the world of celebrities is hooked since then.

Justin Bieber:
His Instagram is covered and he's probably the largest hoverboarder on the planet.
fan of all. He has it all look like a lot of fun, and has the flexibility to make is amazing.
The advantages these devices offer are evident when he is using the devices indoors, outdoors or in parking spaces,

on planes, and almost everywhere and everywhere.

If it's following his pals around the home, playing games of tag, or just chilling

out to test his boarding abilities or even dancing Bieber makes use of these in every way he can.

Situation and is among the self-balancing hoverboards that truly represent self-balancing.

Chris Brown:

One of the greatest dancers is incredibly talented in his own self-balancing

hoverboard. Chris Brown has been pictured and videoed in bars and

club, playing pool or simply exploring the vastness that is his home.

If you're looking for some proof of just how cool these self-balancing scooters are

If you are looking for a new place to hang out, take a look at C-Breezy.

Ivana Korab:

One of the world's most popular models and actresses is amazing

training her hoverboard skills with her model buddies high in Hollywood

Hills. She can make everything look more sexy, and is the perfect spokesperson for the trendy, fashionable, and cutting-edge design of the self-balancing scooter.

Karim Benzema:

The off-season is a literal one, Karim Benzema has decided to give his rest to the next level.

Level using his hoverboard to move about his home, or even cooking while riding it.

Perhaps self-balancing sports aren't too far from your doorstep?

Chapter 9: Drop Shipping

Drop shipping is a method of transferring goods that doesn't really have any inventory at all. You collaborate with a warehouse, wholesaler or other more of a seller. You sell your products through eBay, Amazon, or your own site. You receive payment and then give the customer's information to drop shippers. You "blind ship" which means that there's no trace on their packaging labels, or marketing materials. This means your customer believes that the item was shipped by you.

The margin you earn represents the distinction between the amount you paid the drop-shipper and the amount you offered to sell this board's components to your client for. There is no need to hold any inventory, or handle the shipping.

This is an excellent option for those who don't wish to keep inventory in storage or have a large amount of initial capital but margins won't be as great. Drop shippers will charge more as they're doing the job for you.

Affiliate Marketing

Affiliate Marketing is an excellent opportunity to test your skills since it's free. Affiliate marketing implies that you are employed as an affiliate sales representative for an established seller, whether it's Amazon through Amazon Affiliate Program, eBay via the Amazon Affiliate Program, eBay via the eBay Partner Network and as an affiliate for any of a variety of Hoverboard sellers on the internet who are independent. You distribute affiliate links and receive a fee if anyone who clicks on that link is able to access the site and purchases the hoverboard. Commissions range from around 8% to 20 percent. You can get this done at no cost with Social Media, Youtube, and even free blogging websites like Google's Blogger. With the .blogspot domain. You could choose to purchase the domain as well as hosting or even a store building tool like the Ali Plugin that works with Ali Express.

E-Commerce & Retail

A majority of you do not have an existing brick and mortar retailer, and therefore you'll probably be looking to engage in the world of e-commerce. This could mean selling your products on eBay, Amazon, or your own website , like an Shopify website, although there's millions of plug-and-play stores and shopping carts available.

In the majority of e-commerce sites and not like drop shipping, you purchase and keep all of the items you own. It will take some money to begin but you'll make more profit than drop shipping because you'll get better pricing purchasing in bulk, as opposed to drop shippers who purchase one board at one time. Furthermore, because drop shippers do the actual shipping they will charge more in comparison to buying your inventory in bulk.

For the select few who own a retail store that is a cellphone repair shop or mall kiosk where you sell items out of your bricks and mortar store and receive a higher cost than someone who is online or selling it on Craigslist. This doesn't mean that it's not possible to make money "hustling" in your local area. In the six months leading up to Christmas, I sold more than 1,000 hoverboards online, through local classified websites like Bookoo, Craigslist, Offer Up 5 Miles and various other online applications.

It's true that there were many dealers selling Hoverboards due to the high market demand and profit were more than drugs. Believe it or not.

Wholesaling

This is for who have a substantial budget to invest in your venture, or have having a strong relationship with another warehouse or importer who can store your inventory.

Wholesale is selling to resellers. Instead of selling directly to the final user who actually uses the device, you're going be selling to sellers who resell in stores and on eBay local or on Craigslist. Wholesalers will have lower profits since your customers need an amount of "meat off the bone" or "meat on the bone" or room to earn a profit. Because they purchase in bulk, they can benefit from bulk or wholesale pricing.

However, I think that whole-sale selling to me is the best option, as you're doing not have to deal with 100 customers who will complain about problems with their boards. Customers are resellers, and the issues of retail customers are their responsibility to address.

Another advantage of wholesaling is that instead of selling a single board at a given time to an individual, you can sell 10 20-50, 20-50, perhaps even hundreds of boards one single person at a. While the margins are less, you will earn more because of the quantity of boards you sell.

Parts & Repair

Selling spare parts to fix hoverboards, and also offering repair services is booming. The profits on parts are extremely high, and because of the popularity of the industry, many Chinese manufacturers aren't looking to market their products, but prefer to keep the parts to make more boards. This is why there aren't many people who can find parts or make parts for purchase. You can earn a lot of money not just in parts, but in the actual repair work also.

Most of the time, those working on repairs are working in the field of repair of cellphones. They have the tools and expertise in electronics. This is why a lot of them have taken on the task to repair hoverboards and drones too.

Repairing hoverboards is a breeze and does not require more than the use of a Phillips head screwdriver as well as an assortment of needle nose pliers. Many repairmen currently working are simply watching Youtube videos and getting tips from their peers, and no one is a professional at this point.

Repair costs are astronomical with the cost for a simple task like an repair to a charging port, which is about $80. Repairing the problem will require a part of $3 and five minutes of effort. A more complex repair such as a motherboard or frame might cost $150 to $200. It's likely that to be at some point that spending hundreds of dollars on repairs doesn't seem sensible when you could purchase a brand new motherboard but with some who have paid up to $1500 for theirs, they'd prefer to spend hundreds of dollars to fix it, rather than to throw away it and purchase a new one.

Margins and Profits

The next thing to think about is what do boards cost? What is the price they are sold for? What is the maximum amount you could earn. The industry is evolving rapidly that the numbers I provide today might change the next day.

The boards can be purchased for as little as $70 in China. You'll have to work with the manufacturers. It is necessary decide whether you want you want to ship via ship or by plane and how to go about it. You'll need to know how to fill in customs paperwork and obligations. Also, you must master the art of working with forwarders, unless collecting your cargo at the port by yourself.

On the other hand, you could work with USA wholesalers or warehouses that have already completed all this for you. There is a slight cost more , but you'll have access to boards right away rather than waiting 60-90 days for shipping. If you purchase from the USA according to the size of your order as well as the quantity it is possible to pay anything from $150-$300 at wholesale.

These boards can be purchased for anything from $280 up to as high as $1500. It all depends on a variety of things. Are you selling in a retail store or in a mall? If yes, you'll be able to fetch 400 to $600. You'll be more reliable than an Craigslist seller or an online seller.

Is your city already overflowing with boards? There are cities where you cannot find boards for less than $600 while in others are able to find boards at less than $300 every day long.

How you present your board is also an important impact. Companies such as iOHawk sell identical $200 boards to what everyone other companies are selling, but due to their name and the brand they are selling at up to $1100 or more.

This Program will cover...
This is the introduction for this show. In this program , we will explore the specific aspects of this company...
1. Boards 101 Everything you should be aware of about actual boards
2. Business More details on drop-shipping, wholesale drop-shipping and parts & repair
3. Suppliers - How to locate suppliers and how to negotiate prices
4. Avoiding Scams and Losses It's as simple as avoiding losing money.
5. How to Sell - How to and where do you promote your product
6. My StoryMy Story some tips for you.

7. Links and resources to help your business.
Let's get started!! !

Chapter 10: Today!
In May 2015, in May of 2015, Guinness World Records recognized the "hoverboard" to refer to the device operated by feet. The record was held from Catalina Alexandru Duru, a Canadian who took an controlled flight with the "hoverboard," that looked quite similar to tiny fans with curved blades in a flight of 905 feet and 2 inches at Lake Ouareau, in Canada. The interview with The National, published on YouTube recently, revealed the fact that Mr.
Duru is still working to improve his hoverboard.

Lexus International
On the 24th of June, Lexus International completed its fourth film "Slide" that was a look at the development of a hoverboard prototype. The development was completed in 18 months and comprised the efforts of researchers of IFW Dresden and evico GmbH. It was not just about the technology used in the board, it was also about the magnetic fields and the liquid nitrogen. It was the skate park that was created specifically for this type of hoverboard and

even though they had the top athlete in professional skating, the Ross McGouran it was a constant process of training as if you were mastering new skills. (laura, 2015)

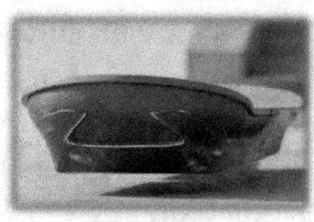

We've come 26 years since we first saw this hoverboard on "Back to the Future: Part 2". This year we are at. (faqs.org 2013,) We're getting closer to achieving the hoverboard. We have started to develop the technology, thanks to research" the most intelligent. The overall picture shows that this is a field that is bursting with new ideas that will surely going to be around for some time!

Chapter 11: Hover Or Glide

Are we seeing an electric scooter or a hoverboard? Well, let"s see. The hoverboard that was portrayed in the films "Back to the Future II" and "Back to the Future III" was modelled on the magnetic field of earth. Marty McFly"s borrowed hoverboard hovered, then floated across the sky. (IMDb 1989) So, there was a bit of floating around, but it was also gliding. What's important is that hoverboards that get close to becoming real has some way to go before they can achieve this dream. Really how do you plan to go on the Hendo Hoverboard in the absence of a copper floor that is specially designed and are able to afford it. In the end, the board cost ten people $10,000.00.

The scientifically-minded would say that we require an opposing metallic (or magnet) to counter the magnetic field on the case of a hoverboard. Oh, how I think I'm Penny in "The Big Bang Theory! "

The initial prototype appeared suspiciously similar to the flux capacitor...but in the end, this was the start of Hendo Hoverboard. Greg Henderson had this first prototype sitting on the table in his home. (Hendo Hover)

It's clear that this isn't something we're likely to see anytime in the near future. Hendo Hover is in the development phase.

Learning to Use the Self-Balancing Scooter

If you were to examine the scooter, one would think that the two-wheeled scooters are quite sophisticated. It's not the reality. All the technology is beneath the two pads you are standing on. There are a variety of self-balancing scooters that are available on the market. Some are heavy, while others cost a lot, and some require time to master according to your balancing capability. There are two types of scooters:

One-wheeled -unicycle

Two-wheeled scooter

Acceleration is the primary factor in the two kinds of scooters. Leaning back or forwards will determine the speed of this direction. Straightening these scooters can slow them down. A different direction of lean is to move left or right. If you slowly move this way you'll notice that this is a fluid movement. Unfortunately, until you locate that "comfort area," that can last up to an hour or more, you could be prone to falling off your scooter often.

They are made to be awe-inspiring for the user. If you're not certain what I mean by that, I'll give you the best explanation I can:

The scooters are equipped with chips under each pad that you use to place your feet. The chips will decide which direction you'd like to go, based upon the pressure that you exert on the foot's parts.

The trick here is the ability to keep your balance. As long as you find your balance, you'll be able to ride any of these rides.

If you are aware of the way your body functions to move you in fluid motion, then you can utilize the scooter to extend of you.

Benefits

The benefits of using these scooters are obvious:

They make use of rechargeable batteries

Convenient

Easy of operation

Low maintenance

Weight limit of 150kg

Advantages

There aren't many of them:

The housing easily scratches

Certain models haven't been evaluated

Trends

The top three countries have shown desire to purchase a two-wheeled vehicle, as per Google Trends.

https://www.google.com/trends/explore#q=hoverboard

With the increase in interest as interest increases, it will be an improved framework for Scooters.

At Xcoot, you will find various ways that are done to meet the needs of regional needs. Xcoot makes it possible to have your scooter delivered within days instead of weeks. Their inventory is available in three central places.

Chapter 12: Inside Out

A fascinating thing was discovered during the journey towards the Patent Office. In fact, you can look up the patent office to check if there's any claims that are similar to yours prior to filing. This is a look at how an auto-balancing two-wheeled vehicle appeared as from inside. It appears that you don't need to go into detail in your sketch, but only with your descriptions. It's enough to demonstrate the relationship between the two sides. It is described in an Abstract at the Patent Office:

The Best Part of all the information you're receiving, it's delightful to find out where the scooter came to us (Thank for the information, Marty McFly - I mean Mr. Gale.)

Xcoot

Let's discuss a bit about this business. Xcoot is comprised of top-rated entrepreneurs from all over the world and is headquartered in Canada. The customer service as well as the return policy and shipping time have helped them stand out from other competitors.

The goal of the business is simple and easy. They aim to provide the best customer service. They provide quick delivery and offer a one-year warranty for the circuit board, and 3 months for hardware. It's a

great way to ensure their product! Now let's take a closer look at the unit itself:
This is the basic characteristics!

A lot of us are done with the shopping for Christmas. Many of us have considered about the "promised" hoverboard. If you're thinking about the idea, there's still an opportunity! The following are facts on the Xcoot as well as the specifics!

A variety of Xcoot
Sure, Xcoot have that. There is plenty of it as well! There's the
Xcoot X2 Series.
Features:
10 inches tires
Clearance increased
This is the larger sister of the Xcoot G2! The tires were enlarged to better withstand the harsh road conditions. The purpose for this design was to aid in achieving performance off-road. This model is not required the use of a manually calibrated remote, or a remote. It comes with an auto-calibration system as that is standard. The maximum speed is around 10 miles an hour, and it can

travel for a distance up to 10 miles without needing to recharge. Four sensors are located underneath the rubber pads. They determine how your feet are set to go. The most safe angle to climb is around 15 degrees, while the weight of the vehicle is around 26lbs.

The Xcoot G3+ is the Last Generation Self-balancing Scooter that has LED and Bluetooth
Features:
Controlled and easy to use
Bluetooth speakers embedded
Connect your smartphone easily to your computer
The scooter is your own extension with its simple design. The built-in Bluetooth speakers will make it enjoyable to drive this bike. You can expect to travel 10-12 miles per hour on this bike, and go up fifteen miles prior to when it has to be charged.

Xcoot G2+ Bluetooth + Led 2 Wheels Self-balancing Scooter
Features:
built on the principle of dynamic balance

You can freely move between forward and reverse, and then stop
Simple operation
Mobility and user-friendliness
One of the best, safest and highest-quality self-balancing scooters that is safe. It comes with a better battery and a more efficient balance system.

Xcoot G3 Self Balancing Scooter
Features:
Based on the concept of dynamic balance
you can move freely forward, backwards and stop
The simplicity of operation
no pollution
User-friendliness
This advanced electrical device turns, as well as the other features that come typical of the Xcoot scooters. It's got a modern design and is capable of climbing at angles of as high as 15 degrees.

The Xcoot G2 Two Wheels Self Balancing Scooter

Features:

Self-balancing electric scooter with high-end quality.
the most popular model
can move forwardor reverse, spin, and stop
Simple operation
no pollution
Mobility and user-friendliness
This is a premium self-balancing electric scooter that is safe similar to the other models. It is similar to an model Xcoot G2Plus Bluetooth + Led Two Wheels self Balancing Scooter, but it doesn"t come with the Bluetooth ability.
That's the basic information about the scooters provided by Xcoot.

Chapter 13: Accessories

Xcoot also has accessories to go with your scooter.

The Wheels

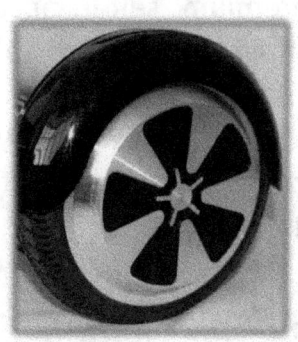

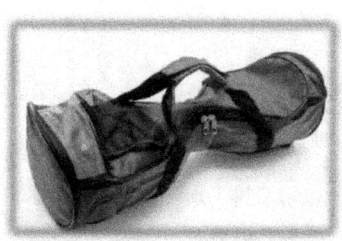

The Bag

Furthermore, it also comes with CE, FCC, and UL approved electric charger. 110V.
Yes, you read it correctly, CE, FCC, and UL Certified!
It gives confidence.

Options
The options are always great! This means that you'll most likely not get the exact as your neighbor across the street. That is, unless that's your goal.
The choices here are colors! Or, I'm talking about patterns! But, I'm talking about both!
XCOOT X2 TWO WHEELERS Self-Blancing Scooter 10 Inches TIRES
The Xcoot G3+ is the Last Generation Self-balancing Scooter equipped with LED and Bluetooth
XCOOT G2+ G2+ LED TWO WHEELS, SELECT BALANCING Scooter
OR

Most of us are finished with our Christmas shopping. We've all thought about the "promised" hoverboard. In case you're still contemplating it, there's an opportunity! These are some facts about Xcoot, along with the specifics!

Chapter 14: The Reality Of Fantasy

We've all heard of The Slide produced by Lexus International, The Hendo Hover initially developed by Greg Henderson, and the Omni Hoverboard which resembles drones created by an engineer Catalin Alexandru Duru. The latter set records in Guinness World Record. The next question to be asked is who will cross the end first.

The Slide was created to create a series of automobile commercials. They hired a team of scientists to aid in their series of commercials. The commercial, or "project" which they've described it the result of their efforts to communicate their design philosophy and to demonstrate their knowledge in creating

Examining Our Reality

What is it that we want when we say that we want a hoverboard, now that there are some on the horizon? Is it just the idea that they can exist and work similar to what we expect? There are a lot of expectations if you compare the hoverboard that Marty McFly was drifting around on with reality today.

McFly's Hoverboard:

Compact enough to easily carry
Intuitive enough for ease of use
Small enough for easy storage, and
No assembly required (strapping in)

Does that remind you of anything? Aside from the unavailable „Slide," we are out of options for anything that truly resembles a hoverboard. I look at that list and I see that it has Xcoot written all over it!

Xcoot Gyroscooters:

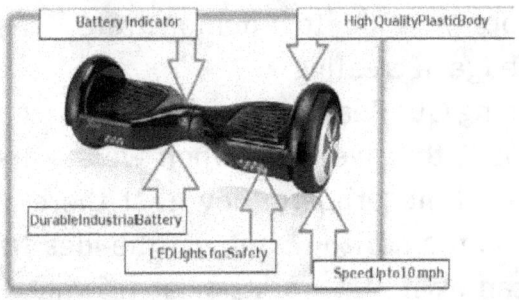

Compact enough to carry in its" own bag
Intuitive enough for ease of use
Small enough for ease of storage
No assembly required (strapping in)

Okay! That definitely puts things into perspective! Besides, If we have to wait for a
"real" hoverboard to come out, well, let's not go there right now!

What we know is this:
The Xcoot is more affordable than any "hoverboard" will ever be
The Xcoot is durable enough for young and old alike
The Xcoot makes a great gift
The Xcoot has a guarantee on their products
The Xcoot is constantly improving their product line.

The colors are great, the models are better. When you ride these Xcooters, it's as if they are an extension of you. Your brain tells your body, and your body tells the Xcooter. It can't get any simpler than that!

Some may view this as a toy, and they are right if they buy it for that purpose.

However, the Xcoot is more than just a toy! It is a sensible way to get around when you are running errands at work or taking your lunch break. It can carry you for a quick trip down the block to your local grocery for a few things you didn't notice, your last big grocery trip. Yes, you can actually carry a grocery bag if you are within your Xcooter's weight limit.

What Does the Future Hold?

For now, we are looking at the Omni Hoverboard going into production sometime after 2017. That's after Catalin Alexandru Duru secures a patent and develops his hoverboard to fly longer than 1.5 minutes. (Russon, 2015) The Hendo Hover is working on a design to slim their model down, but it will only be able to be used "in a special purpose-built conductive rink."

From Mary-Ann Russon's article, Omni Hoverboard: Canadian inventor still refining his Guinness Record-breaking flying propeller device

There are so many drawing and concepts on the internet concerning what a hoverboard should or could look like in the future. Our ability to build them without the restrictions of confining them to a specific surface has eluded our engineers and scientists to this point. Unless we can harness the use of an air- based hoverboard, which would just seem bulky with the need for a motor, it just seems impossible to give us the „Marty McFly" version for which we had hoped.

Our Future is ours to Decide

When and if we ever get to the point that we have a hoverboard that rivals the version in movie Trilogy Back to the Future, I am sure that it will be spread everywhere. There will not be a soul on this earth that will not be aware of the greatest „peace effort" ever made for humanity. In the meantime, we need and want what there is to be had to be happy here and now. That is just human nature.

Chapter 15: Motivation

Mental Meltdown
You're waking up out of bed, 7:00am sharp on a cold December morning. The entire week you've been motivated about becoming a better snowboarder and leading up to today you've made the conscious decision to wake up early, put your snowboarding gear on, grab your equipment, and head straight down to the superpipe to work on your riding technique and mechanics. But now that the day has finally arrived... you realize that it's Saturday, it's cold, your body is sore from yesterday's practice session, and you're just way too warm and comfortable in your bed at the moment to get up and start your workouts. You hit snooze on the alarm and go back to sleep.

What happen to the overflowing amounts of Motivation you had?

Now let's not get carried away, athletes go through these situations all the time and under certain circumstances it's perfectly okay to get some extra rest. After all the grind of a competitive season brings along a lot of stress on the body that requires some recovery and recuperation time. It only becomes a problem when skipping workouts and not following through with your commitments becomes a habit. And unfortunately this is very, and I mean very, common. Just take a listen to some of the promises your friends and peers make when summer time comes around… "I'm going to lose 20 pounds and get my body summer ready… I'm going to diet and eat nothing but fruits and vegetables for the next two weeks… I'm going to wake up early every day and go to the gym."

Fast forward to a few months later and guess what? Absolutely nothing has changed! No diet, no weight loss, and of course no early morning gym sessions. To get to the point, without a true sense of motivation it becomes extremely difficult to get things done. And when you're an aspiring athlete this makes all the difference. To become successful on the snow it's crucial that you identify what your underlying motivation is so that you can feed off of it and use it to fuel your efforts.

Definition & Examples

Motivation: your "reason", your "why" of what you practice for and what you work hard for.

Example

1. "I'm staying late after practice today to work on my indie grab." Why am I staying late? Because I want to be a better snowboarder than my older brother. So my motivation is beating and performing better than my older brother.

Little Known Fact: Motivation as a whole goes a whole lot deeper, and here's a quick breakdown. There are actually two different types of motivation... Intrinsic Motivation and Extrinsic Motivation.

Intrinsic Motivation: motivation that comes from within you or from inside of you.

Example

1. "I have a passion and a love for snowboarding. I don't need any extra attention from people or any special prizes to keep snowboarding, I simply enjoy being part of the sport."

Extrinsic Motivation: motivation that comes from something outside of you.
1. "I like to snowboard because it makes my dad really happy. Also, for every competition that I win I get a crisp $20 bill, this keeps me driven to perform my best.

            Vs $$
Intrinsic   Extrinsic

The Game Plan
Simple distinction right? If you didn't understand the difference between the two types please take a moment and re-read both definitions and examples again. Now, you might be wondering which type of motivation is best for maximizing your talents and efforts? And if you guessed Intrinsic Motivation, you are Correct. Here's why.

When your motivation comes from within you, you don't need some external reward or some type of trophy to work hard and give it your all. It's just something that comes natural to you, and you feel a burning desire inside of you to continue to push yourself. You have a passion and a love for snowboarding, and if you receive anything along the way it's nice to get the recognition but it's not necessary for you to continue to be driven. And the truth is that this is the way most really successful snowboarders maintain high levels of performance. When you're watching your favorite athletes on TV this is difficult to notice because of course they are under the spot light and have all the attention from fans, but what you don't see is the thousands and thousands of hours of practice that go on behind the scenes. And it's no surprise that the best athletes are the same ones who are last to leave the training grounds, despite them already knowing they are better than everyone else.

Now on the other hand, when an athlete is Extrinsically Motivated, they may find success in the beginning... but what eventually ends up happening is their motivation starts to slowly fade away which only leads to the athlete "burning out." If you're not familiar with the term Burn Out, it's simply a term used to describe the physical and mental exhaustion of an athlete. Why does this happen? Well, this type of athlete works hard also, but only works hard for the reward, works hard for the trophy, works hard for the scholarship, works hard for the money. Once the athlete acquires these external objects that he/she is motivated in attaining, what's next? What comes after that? What becomes their reason for continued hard work and effort? NOTHING! There aren't any other reasons or desires to want to continue to improve and get better. Since this athlete's sole motivation was to possess that external reward, once it's in their hands they become complacent, comfortable, and un-driven. With that being said, there's no problem with getting recognition for athletic achievement...it's actually something to be extremely proud of and something that should be celebrated. The issue only becomes apparent if you're true underlying goal is to become the BEST.

So what's the take away? In order to be successful on the snow you need to find your true Intrinsic Motivation. Find your Why. Find your reason. And make sure it's something that makes YOU happy, NOT someone else. Keep that fire inside of you burning for as long as possible, because once it's gone it's very hard to get it lit again.

Mental Workout

1. Write down all the reasons why you snowboard. What's your motivation for snowboarding? Is it Intrinsic or Extrinsic?

2. Write down all the reasons why you think you feel motivated one day, and unmotivated the next day. What types of distractions do you have around you? How can you avoid these distractions from getting in the way of your success?

3. Talk to your friends and teammates and see if you can find what drives their motivation. Can you tell who is Extrinsically Motivated and who is Intrinsically Motivated?

Goal-Setting

Mental Meltdown

Imagine this... You wake up from a long nap and find yourself alone in a car with no phone or any type of technology in sight. You're headed on a long road trip to a small town that you know is somewhere to the

North of you but you have no directions as to how to get there. You really have no idea how far this place is or how long it should take you to get there.

What are you to do?

This example is a little far-fetched (as you will probably never be put in this position), but it makes the perfect point: YOU CAN'T REALLY KNOW WHERE YOU'RE GOING WITHOUT A CLEAR ROADMAP! And a goal is exactly that, a roadmap to reach your desired level of success. For some odd reason however, many of today's youth athletes really have no desire to create clear and concise goals. Which leads to the questions... Where are you going? How will you get there? When will you get there? What do you need in order to arrive on time?

The Best Athletes know what they want, they understand exactly what it will take to get there, and they know how long it will take them to get there. It's not a very complicated process to understand, but there are some key factors you need to be aware of in terms of learning proper goal setting techniques. Once you get these strategies down, you'll be light years ahead of your peers and will drastically improve your chances of success!

Definition & Examples

Goal- the end result of something you are targeting or trying to accomplish.

Example

1. "My goal is to be the best snowboarder I can be."

Most of the goals you set for yourself are very likely similar to the example given above. Really simple, really generic, and straight to the point. But there's a huge problem with setting goals this way. What's the problem? These types of goals never get accomplished! They never get accomplished because there's no way of measuring any type of progress. Setting a very vague goal doesn't give you the ability to track whether or not you're taking steps forward, taking steps backwards, or staying in the exact same place. The simple solution to this requires the athlete to become more specific, which leads us to our next point…there are two categories when it comes to goal setting: short term goals and long term goals.

Long Term Goal- your main objective/target. (big picture)

Short Term Goal- checkpoints that need to be reached in order to accomplish your long term goal. (small scope)

Example

1. "Two months from now I want to increase the amount of weight I can squat at my max by 40 pounds, that's my long-term goal. In order to do that I need to increase the amount of weight I can squat at my max by 20 pounds every month, which breaks down into an increase of about 5 pounds per week, those are my short-term goals. In order to increase the amount of weight I can squat at my max by 5 pounds every week I'm going to do squats every other day after practice and I'm going to keep track of how many sets I do as well as how much weight I can add to the bar (even more precise short term goals)." The more precise you get, the better.

Week 1
Monday   Tuesday   Wednesday   Thursday   Friday

3 sets of 4 reps at 140lbs   3 sets of 4 reps at 140lbs   2 sets of 3 reps at 145lbs

Overall= increase of 5lbs

Week 2

Monday   Tuesday   Wednesday   Thursday   Friday

2 sets of 3 reps at 145lbs   2 sets of 4 reps at 145lbs   3 sets of 2 reps at 150lbs

Overall= increase of 5lbs

Week 3

Monday   Tuesday   Wednesday   Thursday   Friday

2 sets of 3 reps at 150lbs   3 sets of 2 reps at 150lbs   1 set of 2 reps at 155lbs

Overall= increase of 5lbs

Week 4

Monday   Tuesday   Wednesday   Thursday   Friday

1 set of 2 reps at 150lbs   2 sets of 2 reps at 150lbs   1 set of 1 rep at

160lbs
Overall= increase of 5lbs

The Game Plan

Okay let's quickly recap. You need to set a long term goal (destination) along with short term goals (specific directions) to help you reach your target level of success. Simple. now let's take it one step further. Whenever you set a long term or short term goal you need to make sure that it's not Too Easy, but not Impossibly Difficult. The level of difficulty that every goal should fall between is right around the moderately difficult category. Take a look at the spectrum that follows.

Goal Setting Level of Difficulties

Too Easy- Not at all challenging for you

Moderately Easy- Only a little challenging for you

Neutral- An even balance between easy and challenging for you

Moderately Difficult- Challenging and pushes your Limits

Too Difficult- Overly challenging and difficult to notice any real progress

The magic formula lands in the moderately difficult category for the simple reason that these types of goals challenge you and test your limits but also give you a certain sense of belief that you can accomplish what you've set out to accomplish. Let's consider the other side of the coin. When a goal is too easy it doesn't challenge or motivate you which leads to boredom, and when a goal is extremely difficult it's really hard for you to see any results or progress. Without seeing any results or progress your confidence is shot down to the ground, and will eventually lead to you quitting or giving up. That's the last thing we want.

Finally, something that you absolutely must remember from now on every time you set a goal should incorporate the following characteristics. The acronym is SMART. Here's what it stands for:

Specific: every goal you set must be very specific, clear, and concise.

Measurable: every goal you set must have some measurable aspect to it. If you're looking to become faster you can time yourself, if you want to get stronger you can keep track of how much weight you're lifting.

Action-oriented: every goal should require you to take action whether physically or mentally.

Realistic- as we mentioned before your goals need to be realistic (in the moderately difficult category, not impossibly difficult or incredibly easy).

Timely- all goals need to have a deadline, some sort of time frame to ensure you're doing everything you can to reach your target.

And there you have it, the Proper Goal Setting Techniques. By incorporating all facets: Long Term Goals, Short Term Goals, The Goal Setting Difficulty Spectrum, and SMART…you are equipped to improve your performance to a very high level at a very quick pace. And remember, as you begin to accomplish the goals you've set things will become easier and easier for you, allowing you to modify your goals as you go which will only make you that much better as an athlete.

Mental Workouts

1.   Begin now, write down 3 long term goals you want to accomplish.

2.   Develop a plan and a series of short term goals of how you will accomplish those 3 long term goals. Remember to keep track, whether daily, weekly, or monthly.
Mental Imagery

Mental Meltdown
There's nothing like watching one of those classic and exciting snowboarding movies. From Back in Black, to The Community Project, to Run to the Hills, The Art of Flight, The Fourth Phase, and list can go and on... There's just something special about watching a movie about the sport you love that motivates you to get back on your snowboard and work your tail off! This may be in part due to the fact that so many of us consciously or unconsciously put ourselves in the role of the main characters in the movie. We take a ride on the emotional roll-a-coaster the film is portraying... we feel the pain, we feel the anguish, we feel the frustration, and at the end we feel the triumph and success when the movie

characters pull it together and get the Win in the face of Adversity.

And in actuality, this exact process is a lot how Mental Imagery (also known as Visualization) works! Mental Imagery is like having a movie in your head, and simply hitting Play on the DVD player whenever you're ready to watch it.

Unlike the movies however, in real life things don't always end the way you'd want them to end. For example, after having a bad round or not performing up to your standards you may think back and begin to run all the costly mistakes you made during the course of the competition or across the entire season. You visualize yourself not getting enough air on your jumps, forgetting your routine, not landing properly, getting frustrated, getting yelled at, being made fun of, and losing your position on the team despite all your hard work and effort. And in doing so you get yourself into a huge "funk" which is the exact opposite of what you wanted in the first place! In order to avoid this from happening, it's crucial you realize that the images you play in your head have an enormously powerful impact on your snowboarding performance. Learning the proper way to utilize Mental Imagery is vital, and it's important you use it as an advantage instead of as a pitfall so your abilities can reap the positive benefits.

Definition & Example
Mental Imagery (Visualization)- using your thought processes and imagination to create very detailed images and pictures in your mind. These images can be of past experiences or future moments in the way you would like them to play out.

Example

1. I'm at the top of the slope ready to practice my barrel roll backflip. I close my eyes and imagine preparing to board down. I begin my approach, the crowd is roaring, I can feel the pressure, but I'm confident. I bend my knees, gain the necessary speed, and launch off the ramp. I throw my head back sending me into my rotation, locate my landing spot, and stick the landing like a pro. The crowd goes wild, my teammates are jumping up and down with excitement, I can feel the adrenaline running through my veins, a perfect score!

LIGHTS….CAMERA…. ACTION!!

The Game Plan

If you're aspiring to be a great snowboarder at some point, then you've most definitely closed your eyes and dreamed about experiencing massive success during competition… about landing high difficulty tricks… about making incredible come from behind victories…. and gaining all the respect from your friends and peers. And it's perfectly normal, all great athletes do it regardless of the sport they participate in. What's important however is to realize that the way you process these mental images must be done in an effective and efficient manner. Believe it or not, there is a certain science to it. Here is a check list of components you need to use in order to apply Mental Imagery to your snowboarding career and maximize your potential.

Before working on your jumps, before boarding into a half pipe, before participating in a competition, anything that requires a specific skill set or process, take ten minutes and just visualize yourself being successful. Visualize yourself correctly executing every move, every movement, and every step. Imagine perfectly landing each and every trick attempt during your routine, being so flawless that no one can match your performance, being so smooth that you make it look easy for anyone who's watching. You're just overflowing with confidence and can handle anything that comes your way. Along this process however, it's important that you be very, and I mean very detailed and specific on the pictures you're running through your mind. Like I mentioned earlier, it should be like playing a movie in your head.

You must use all your senses: touch, sight, smell, hear, taste. As you begin to learn how to incorporate all your senses, you will start to notice that you will progressively feel more and more as if you were presently in the moment you are imagining. And this is what we're aiming for. Because you're envisioning vivid and detailed mental pictures your brain begins to release the exact same chemicals and signals throughout your body as if you were actually in that moment. This will allow you to experience the same emotional responses and phenomenon's you would have as if it were happening in real time, thus allowing you to prepare in advance and give you the feeling as if "You've been there before" when that moment finally arrives.

Example:

Let's say that during last week's giant slalom competition you weren't able to turn the corners properly which costed you precious seconds off the clock. You know you can snowboard much better, so before this week's competition you take ten minutes and visualize yourself successfully executing your routine and turning the corners perfectly…. "I'm at the starting line, I can feel the cold breeze brushing across my face, I can hear the crowd cheering on the other boarder, I can smell and almost taste the popcorn coming from the snack bar, but my eyes are locked in on the course. The gate opens up…and I go through my usual routine…I get a great push off the starting position…lean forward and bend my knees, stay balanced and centered, flex my ankles and lock my edge, and perfectly carve around the first marker." And repeat this same process again and again turn after turn and carve after carve...elevating your confidence each step of the way.

Learning how to become efficient in the use of mental imagery can be very challenging at times because it's not something that will give you immediate results. So it's important to remember that just like every other skill you've ever learned, you only get better with dedicated time and practice. When you were a baby and first started to learn how to walk it didn't just take you 1 day, it took you weeks, even months to learn how to execute every movement correctly. Don't get discouraged or frustrated in your beginning stages of mental imagery practice, even if you feel like it's not working. Keep practicing, keep getting better, and in time your skill set will in fact positively benefit.

Mental Workout

1. Follow the steps given in the last few paragraphs. Take a skill you want to be better at, and before practicing or even during practice, envision yourself being successful. Picture yourself doing everything right. Remember to be very specific, think

about all the steps, all the movements, and everything around you.

2. Once you start learning how mental imagery can work for you, start developing a routine. Maybe there's a quiet place that you can visit, a song you can play on your ipod, or a certain time of day when visualizing is more effective for you (in the morning when you wake up, or at night before you go to sleep). Repeat that routine as often as possible. Write your routine down.

Thought Suppression

Mental Meltdown
You're boarding down the ramp at extremely high speeds with time running down on the clock. It's the end of the third round and all you need to do is perform a solid trick and stick the landing to put yourself in a great position to come away with a win and secure a spot in the final round. But...as you approach the ramp and take flight...you notice you don't have the speed needed to complete the trick you were going to attempt which breaks your

concentration for a split second. You go for the trick anyway and you end up being unable to stick the landing...just missing your mark by inches and losing your balance causing you to fall. You end up losing the round and losing your chance to make it to the championship round. On the car ride home you can't help but have the same recurring thought run clear across your mind...

"I DON'T WANT TO THINK ABOUT IT ANYMORE!"

It happens to the best of us...all we want to do is bury that unforgiving memory into the deepest and darkest crevice of our mind and lock it away forever and ever...never to be seen again. We want to get as far away as possible from those traumatizing and overwhelming feelings of despair, frustration, and disappointment.

This type of thought process is called Thought Suppression and it's exactly what many athletes engage in after a poor performance. But is Thought Suppression an effective strategy? Is Thought Suppression the best approach to overcoming a bad performance? What is the result of suppressing your thoughts? Well, in reality Thought Suppression is mentally one of the worst things you can possibly do when it comes to trying to elevate your athletic performance. It's really a lot like not studying before a big test, you're simply setting yourself up for failure.

Definition and Examples
Thought Suppression- attempting to stop thinking about a certain idea, or trying to stop certain thoughts from running through your mind.
Example
1. Let's further consider the same example given in the previous section. You've missed your chance to advance to the final round and are now on a very long car ride home. You continue to have the same recurring thought "DON'T THINK ABOUT IT!!!"

The next day is here and you're trying not to think about the incident. To help you trying something new... each when those thoughts of your missed landing come back into your mind You try to distract yourself from those thoughts by focusing on other thoughts that are detached and not connected. You contemplate the delicious tastes of your favourite food...you contemplate your coming family vacation...and you contemplate the way your new Jordan shoes will fit your. (things which usually make to feel more comfortable)

What do you think What? Here's where things become somewhat confusing, as the first thing that happens is that the painful memories of missing your landing gets linked to happy memories of your favourite foods, your family trip and the brand recently purchased Jordan shoes. That means every when you think of these enjoyable memories...your mind goes back to the moment you missed your landing!

It's hard to understand what this is all about initially however it's a widespread phenomenon in psychology referred to as the Rebound Effect.

Rebound Effect of Thought SuppressionAs you attempt to shut down the thought (not to think about it) but you find yourself being thinking about it for a longer time. Your mind gets absorbed in thinking about the exact thing you do not want to be thinking about!

T

The Game Plan

As it's a concept that is contradictory Let's discuss it in greater depth. Memory functions in your brain is by making connections between items or concepts. For instance, if you hear someone say "dog" what immediately occurs in your mind? It's likely that you start thinking about the terms "paws or bark, bite and even fur." The more strong the bonds are formed between connected objects or concepts and the more likely that you will be able to remember these particular memories. Because your mind can't differentiate between undesirable memories and pleasant ones and pleasant memories, when you're blocking your thoughts and trying to replace a painful memory with a positive one, you're in fact creating a connection between both. This is crucial to know whether you're a snowboarder or an athlete generally because "DON'T think about it" is often exactly the opposite of what you want to achieve. purpose is...which will be to overcome your embarrassing performance or moment. This leads to you to ask.. If not thinking about it does not bring about the desired outcome What do you do to assist you in getting over your mistake?

There are numerous options available, but one is different from other options ....and it's known as the Mindfulness method. You may have heard the concept of Mindfulness at the beginning of your career, or maybe even seen it on Television Professional athletes are beginning to realize the potential of Mindfulness. Kevin Pearce (former Olympic snowboarder who suffered a brain injury during in training to compete at the Olympics) has become a well-known person who teaches mindfulness techniques to young athletes to enhance their performance in competition. Many books and articles have been written on mindfulness, and numerous research studies are being conducted to demonstrate its benefits that have been acknowledged by sports organizations across the globe. To be clear though... mindfulness is just a term to define a state of mind that allows you to feel any thoughts and decide to look at them with a non-judgmental attitude. You can accept that thoughts aren't necessarily negative or positive, but just a normal part that happens in human existence. Mindfulness lets you live the present in its entirety and allows you to take whatever happened. Particularly in the case of snowboarding, it is important to recognize that there are fluctuations and ups and downs, and no athlete is immune to this, no matter how skilled they may be. It is inevitable that mistakes will occur and you should not let you allow them to derail you while you attempt to progress in your career. In the event you are prone to Thinking Suppression, you must be conscious and incorporate more of an Mindfulness approach to your thinking process. Your snowboarding experience as an athlete is bound to become more enjoyable and productive.

M

Ental Workout

1. If you're ever participating in a contest, make sure you keep track of your thoughts that affect your performance in a negative way. Record these thoughts below.

2. Look at your list above. Do you think these thoughts are a result of negative experience that you've experienced previously? Explain.

3. How can you apply the Mindfulness approach right away to keep you from repressing your thoughts?

Anxiety About Competition

Mental Meltdown
You've been waiting all year for the moment to come. It's an hour away. Everything you've put into throughout the season is now at stake. All those hours of training and early morning workouts, and late night film sessions the sweat, the blood and tears, the suffering, agony and defeat...all culminating in this moment. The championship round of the tournament.

What's your mood? Sweaty palms? Are you experiencing knots or butterflies inside your belly? Are you struggling to stretch out and loosen up? Gazing out at the spectators and realizing the number of people watching you play? Do you feel the tension to win?

Whether you're in a youth league or in the pros... young or old...a rookie or a veteran...competitive anxiety is experienced by every and all athletes at some point in their careers. Although experiencing some anxiety before a match is common, it can happen at occasions that athletes get so overwhelmed that anxiety takes over their thinking process, which results in an extreme underperformance.

What exactly is this thinking process? First of all the anxiety that cripples you is usually the result of internal fear. The fear takes control of the mind of the athlete, and the thoughts that trigger fear produce fearful feelings and these fearful feelings can lead to fearful behavior. This cycle is extremely difficult to break out of. However, with the proper attitude and training you can minimize the possibility of having high levels of anxiousness in the times which are most important for you as well as your teammates.

D

definition and examples

Competitive Anxiety- the anxious sensation you feel prior to an event, at crucial moments during the contest or even after a race. It is usually an idea in your head that is "expecting" to be the case, and this specific event causes you to very nervous.

Alongside Competitive Anxiety There are two common outcomes: Fear of Failure and the fear of choking under Pressure.

1. Fear of Failure: an enormous fear of risking with your life, the fear of making mistakes and a fear of moving beyond your familiar area, fear being unsuccessful, fear losing and the consequences that might be the result.

Example

a. Sometimes , at the conclusion of the practice, coaches choose one of their boarders to complete an obstacle course within a predetermined duration of time. If the player is able to complete the course within the time allocated, the practice for the day will be completed. If the participant cannot make the required time, the whole team must stay to conduct conditioning exercises. Do you happen to be the one who takes the initiative to finish the course and then fall back and not want to face the burden? Are you scared of the consequences that could come when you fail to finish the course in time?

2. Choking (Choking under pressure)is when you are not doing as well as you usually are. When snowboarding, choking in crucial moments is typically linked to losing to a less skilled opponent, and losing in a contest with a large lead, then giving up to the opposition, and "shrinking" or avoiding in the most critical moment of a contest.

T

The Game Plan

So , what do you do to keep anxiousness about competing from destroying your skiing career? Do you know how to ensure that you no ever again be afraid of failing that is preventing you from achieving your goals? And how can you prevent being a victim in the times when it is most important both for your and the team you work with?

One of the first things you have to be able to identify what makes you anxious and what creates fear in you and then what is it that makes you perform less. The most frequent causes that can lead to higher levels of anxiety about competing might be a shock to your family, friends or even teammates and coaches. What causes this? A lot of young athletes are focused on what the opinions of other people could be in the event that they put in poor performance. For instance, what would your peers discuss at school the following day when you blow a massive lead in the competition yesterday? How upset could your family feel in the event that you fell asleep in the best trick contest and missed the chance to advance? How anxious would you feel going to practice the next day and realize that your teammates and coaches are furious that you didn't remember your routine and were not able to perform it? If any of these scenarios have popped through your thoughts during the last few years, do not to worry, you're certainly not the only one! It's crucial to remember that neither of these scenarios are actual! This is right, I'll say it once more, they're not actually happening. They're all thoughts that cross your mind and stem from...yup you've got it right... fear. If you put aside the negative consequences and focused on the task in hand the emotion response within your body would totally change. This will in turn decrease the amount of anxiety that you suffer from.

Sometimes snowboarders suffer from stress, anxiety and fear of failing and even choke under pressure because of an unfavorable experience before. This is a different in that when the same situation occurs and those thoughts come back to haunt you, which brings with them all negative emotions and thoughts that had previously pushed the athlete to perform poorly. But there's a distinction to be made in this regard that will surely alter the outcomes for those athletes. And here it is...Instead of thinking of past failures as obstacles, as insurmountable mountains, as impossible challenges...athletes should instead think of those failures as opportunities to learn, as chances to correct a mistake, as a second wind to blow past the competition. By doing this, they will alter their thought process, which is what makes the difference. It's all about the perspective. It's only when you are willing to let yourself be lost. Every single failure you face is a learning experience that you can learn from and being able to transfer that experience to your present situation is essential to achieve the level of success that you are so eagerly seeking.

Chapter 16: Self-Talk

Mental Meltdown

"How did I become so foolish? Why didn't I do this move when I had the opportunity? Why am I continuing to train even when it seems that I'm not improving? Perhaps I should stop?"

The questions above are the moment when an athlete is hit by a brick wall and begins to judge themselves in a way that is not productive. When it's the result of boarding an unlucky round or making a mistake on you turn or making an error in practice...athletes in all sports have these situations as they're often inevitable, but difficult to conquer. In general, very little is performed by trainers and coaches to rectify these self-reflections that creates a huge obstacle for an athlete to acknowledge that they have a problem and an unforgivable behavior that's not in their advantage. This unwelcome problem and behavior is an immediate negative effect on the athletic performance of the athlete.

This problem can be addressed through the development of the mental ability (yes it's a talent) self-talk. And , contrary to what you might believe...Self-Talk has been proven to be a effective psychological tool which is utilized by the most accomplished athletes around the world. There are some important distinctions it is important to start by delving into what exactly Self-Talk means and divide it into two distinct types.

D

Definitions and examples

Self-Talk: talking or speaking to yourself in public or through your thoughts.

Simple. To make sure that athletes aren't judging themselves negatively as well as their performances, two kinds of self-talk have become popular.

Positive Self-Talk: tell yourself positive phrases, words and affirmations that motivate you and help you stay focused on the goal you want to achieve.

Example

1. When I am preparing to run on the halfpipe, I think to me, "No one can beat me." "I'm far too proficient." "I am able to easily be victorious."

2. "Hard Work is better than Talent when Talent isn't Working at all" is a common quote.

Instructional Self-Talk: letting yourself know the right instructions to ensure you're meeting your expectations.

Example

1. When you try an indy jump, you can say the following to your mind "build momentum, keep your feet at a low level, and remain in the center for the leap. Make a powerful ollie, grasp the edge of the board and then land safely, keeping your weight placed on the edge of your board." Just as your coach will instruct you to perform during your the practice.

T

The Game Plan

It might seem odd to you that small changes in the way you view and react to your personal behavior and outcomes could have significant changes to your performance on the field. However, in reality it is true that words can be extremely powerful and can have a significant influence on the way you perceive the world. Particularly when we begin to think about the best ways to face the challenges of life and how to get through crucial moments in your career and keep pushing the limits even when your tank is full of fumes...self-talk is a great resource. One of the best examples is none other then Mark McMorris, Canadian professional snowboarder. If you're unfamiliar with his story, in early March 2017 while riding on an off-trail spot located in British Columbia he accidentally crashed into a tree with a high speed. After the accident, he suffered fractured jaw, a broken left arm, ruptured the spleen unstable pelvic fracture, fractures of the ribs along with a collapsed left lung...Mark himself was astonished that to have survived the crash. It was horrifying. As you might imagine, it's been a very long journey towards recovery, which has put him through physical and psychologically.

As you could guess...one of the most important mental abilities he's relying on to aid him in his recovery process has been self-talk! If you're able to read about his journey, take the time to do it as it's an inspiring read. It's been reported that at certain times, the self would say to his self

"I'm extremely content to be alive and be recuperating "... "I'm extremely determined to get this done "... "I'm eager to returning to the slopes, that's my current focus." Then, slowly, his thinking process began to take in a positive direction... He changed his mind from thinking he had suffered an injury that could have ended his career to believing he was in the potential to resume snowboarding at a high level. In the present, he's progressing through his rehabilitation program and is considering an opportunity to return during the 2018 Olympics in South Korea, in which it is believed that he's one of the most likely to be a winner in the large air sports.

If you are interested in the idea of positive or instructive self-talk, my suggestion is to employ both and not one over one over the other. If you can develop each of these mental abilities, you will gain a significant advantage over your competition. This will help you improve your ability to remain focus, which is an outdated skill in today's sporting world. It is also suggested that you begin to develop your own "script." This is a written script you can utilize whenever you're feeling like you require an extra boost to your confidence or to help you get over any bump you're facing. The script you create can be derived from anywhere, or you could develop it on your own or search "Motivational Quotes" and you'll come across a variety of short sentences that are created to keep you motivated and focused. There's one thing for sure that you'll face a variety of challenging situations during your time as a snowboarder. There's no any doubt. It's essential to make sure that when challenges do occur and are thrown at you, it's your turn to tackle them using the tools that will allow you to face and conquer.

Exercise for the MENTAL

1. Spend some time writing down 10 phrases, words and affirmations that keep you focus. You can make use of anything you've seen in a film or read in a magazine or heard in a story It could be something that a friend of yours has said to you, or advice from a teacher or any other source you'd like to. Mix it to make it your own.

_____

2. Imagine yourself in a competitive scenario and think about how you can apply

self-instruction. Record some examples of what you could tell yourself. Record as many instances as you can.

Zones of Maximum Performance

Mental Meltdown
Consider a moment to think about the time you watched your most loved snowboarder perform at a high-level performance. It could be anything from Shaun White winning competition after competition and Gretchen Bleiler landing the first Crippler 540 at the course of a competition, or Billy Morgan landing the first ever quad cork in the 1800s, (just to mention a couple) There are numerous instances which have left the audience stunned and in awe. They seem to perform incredible tricks flawlessly every time. each adjustment appears to boost them to higher levels of skill and ability and it appears like they're ten levels ahead of the rest. What do these amazing feats have in common, regardless of the person doing them? In any after-competition interviews you'll definitely hear them saying...

"I was in the ZONE."

Attaining that "Zone" is among the most sought-after goals of every athlete, regardless of the sport the athlete is playing. It's a mindset that allows everything flowing in your direction and everything seems to be effortless and natural. When it comes to snowboarding, many athletes talk about the joy of snowboarding as winning in competitions like eating candy from a toddler and each move is effortless and smooth. It's an amazing thing to watch...and wouldn't it be even more thrilling if you, as an athlete could learn how to reach this state of mind? Wouldn't it be amazing to be able to reproduce this effect over and over again? Your snowboarding skills would surely shoot up! Therefore, our aim here is to give you notes that can aid you in determining the place where your zone of performance is in order to be able to apply the skills needed to attain this mental state.

D

Definition and Example

Zone of Optimal Performance - the level of anxiety you excel at reaching the "mental zone" and achieving the state of flow, in

which everything seems to flow effortlessly and you are at the highest level athletically.
Example
1. When Billy Morgan landed his amazing flight of an 1800 quadruple cork backside, it was clear from the beginning that he'd been an individual on a mission. Every time he tried the trick, and failed, it appeared that he grew more confident, smarter, and more determined. There was no way to hinder him from achieving his goal. In post-move interviews, Billy provided some insight as to what he experienced when he completed his famous technique... saying things like "The sensation is hard to explain. "... "You do not feel it because of anything else. It's total happiness and energy." It's almost that he was experiencing an unreal experience since he was so immersed in doing whatever was required to make the trick. And he didn't realize the moment was some of the most amazing moments in the history of snowboarding.

T

He Game Plan

The possibilities for how Billy Morgan was able to achieve one of the most amazing tricks of all time are limitless (since Billy Morgan is one of the few athletes not on earth). But, from a sport psychological perspective, there are a number of things we can look at to help us understand what and how athletes are able to reach a mental zone and a state of flow which allow athletes to play at a high level. One of them is the ability to perform under stress, being able to be relaxed and comfortable and overcome anxiety of making mistakes during the course of a contest.

In time's end, all of the various factors result in one road...Learning to deal with anxiety. Check out the Chart which is below.

The graph above provides an approximate average of the places athletes believe they are performing best with regard to their anxiety levels (nerves). As you can observe (the two most high points) that most athletes are at their peak anxiety level when they have an anxiety self-rating score around 3 or an self-rating score of about 8. Scores that are close to level 3 could be best defined as having moderately "low" anxiety, while scores at or near levels 8 and 9 can be described in the category of slightly "high" stress. All of it comes to individual differences (personality behavior, attitude and more.). What does this mean? It's a sign that some athletes prefer to work at a moderately low level of anxiety since that's the level they are at their best. It's the level at which they are comfortable and at a point that makes them feel confident and where they feel at ease. The same reasoning applies to the others who choose to snowboard with relatively high anxiety levels. It's just a matter perception and your personal preferences.

Let's look at the other end part of the range. What is the reason athletes don't perform very well with self-ratings for low anxiety of 1 or at high anxiety self-ratings of 10? This is the answer...when athletes don't feel nervous even a bit (anxiety self-rating of one) they do not perform well on the snowboard because they're not enthusiastic and aren't driven to perform and they're not fully involved in the sport they're doing. They just perform the routine. Do you think of being a snowboarder in a contest against a 2-year-old's? Sure , you'd be the best snowboarder at the contest but it would also be boring since it isn't a contest! Everyone needs to experience an element of stress to boost our energy and keep us on track. On the other hand when athletes are truly anxious (anxiety rate of 10,) the athletes get anxious, stress them out. Then get stuck at the present moment. Being afflicted with a lot of anxiety in one go usually leads to a decrease in performance athletically. In addition, excessive anxiety can be harmful to overall health and could cause a myriad of mental health issues.

Mental Workout

1. I would like you to think about a time in your life that you were in your absolute best. What was it like? Did you get to a "zone"? Did you feel there was lots of pressure placed on you? How stressed or anxious were you prior to, during, and following the event?

2. Consider a moment where you were at your most pathetic. How did you feel? Did you feel lots of tension on your part? How stressed or nervous were you prior to the event, as well as after the event?

3. Review your answers to questions 1 and 2. Do you see any commonalities between these two questions? Are there any distinct differences? What does this say about you?

4. What are some tips you can do prior to your next event or your next training session to assist you in getting into your optimal zone? Also, visit the internet and study how your top snowboarders. Do you know of any tricks their routines are that could benefit from?

www.ingramcontent.com/pod-product-compliance
Lightning Source LLC
Chambersburg PA
CBHW071838080526
44589CB00012B/1034